Family and Self

Family and Self

Bowen Theory and the Shaping of Adaptive Capacity

Robert J. Noone

LEXINGTON BOOKS
Lanham • Boulder • New York • London

Published by Lexington Books
An imprint of The Rowman & Littlefield Publishing Group, Inc.
4501 Forbes Boulevard, Suite 200, Lanham, Maryland 20706
www.rowman.com

86-90 Paul Street, London EC2A 4NE

British Library Cataloguing in Publication Information Available

Library of Congress Cataloging-in-Publication Data

Names: Noone, Robert J., author.
Title: Family and self : Bowen theory and the shaping of adaptive capacity / Robert J. Noone.
Description: Lanham : Lexington Books, [2021] | Includes bibliographical references and index. | Summary: "In Family and Self: Bowen Theory and the Shaping of Adaptive Capacity, Robert J. Noone examines Murray Bowen's theory of the family and its clinical application"— Provided by publisher.
Identifiers: LCCN 2021033953 (print) | LCCN 2021033954 (ebook) | ISBN 9781793628145 (cloth) | ISBN 9781793628169 (paperback) | ISBN 9781793628152 (epub)
Subjects: LCSH: Family psychotherapy. | Dysfunctional families—Evaluation. | Bowen, Murray, 1913-1990.
Classification: LCC RC488.5 .N66 2021 (print) | LCC RC488.5 (ebook) | DDC 616.89/156—dc23
LC record available at https://lccn.loc.gov/2021033953
LC ebook record available at https://lccn.loc.gov/2021033954

To my life partner Kathy

*To Jamie, Brendan, and Caitlin who have each
so ably managed life's challenges*

*To my parents, Martin Noone and Mae McNulty,
and the remarkable adaptive capacity of the
many generations of my County Mayo families*

Contents

Acknowledgments

This book is the product of my own effort to present Bowen theory, but obviously represents the contributions of many. I am immensely grateful to the following:

Mike Kerr and Dan Papero stand out as among the best of systems thinkers each of whom has contributed to my learning of the family and natural systems over the decades. My colleagues at the Center for Family Consultation, especially Stephanie Ferrera, Carol Moran, and Sydney Reed, who have been fellow travelers in the exploration of family systems. The many faculty at The Bowen Center for the Study of the Family whose ongoing work over the years has contributed to the development of Bowen theory and my learning. There is a network of professional colleagues across the country who also represent an important part in the pursuit of knowledge of the human family and in increasing the awareness of the new paradigm of the family as a natural system. I am grateful to Mark Flinn who afforded me the opportunity to observe and learn from his research in Dominica. I have likewise greatly benefited from the many outstanding scientists who have participated in the annual symposia sponsored by the Georgetown Family Center in Washington and CFC in Chicago.

I have had the privilege of meeting with families in my practice and in community mental health centers for many years. The experience has been central to my learning of the struggles and resilience of families. I have gained much from hearing of their current life challenges and as well as from their multigenerational family histories.

It was my good fortune to have been in contact with Murray Bowen from 1975 until his death in 1990. He was a scientist of the first order. Psychiatrist, researcher, teacher, and coach, he and his work contributed to my life and that of countless others. His observations and conceptualizations of the human family resulted in the development of an original formal theory of the family and human behavior. I hope this book will contribute to the growing awareness of his remarkable achievement and his contribution to a science of human behavior.

Introduction

Family and Self is about the family systems theory of the family developed by Murray Bowen. It is also to a degree about the development of my own effort to gain knowledge about human behavior and my own self. Early in my professional life, after several years of searching, I settled on Bowen theory as the principal conceptual framework in my exploration. This book represents my current understanding of this rich theory and my exploration of the scientific literature which I have found especially relevant to my curiosity about human behavior. While the discovery of the family as a vital element in gaining knowledge about self, I have not included the exploration of my personal family in this book. That journey has been central throughout my adult life and Bowen theory opened a vista into my immediate and multigenerational family which has been extraordinarily enriching. My primary intention in *Family and Self* is the broad scope of the theory and its relevance to a science of human behavior.

Bowen theory is an applicable theory for use in clinical practice and in enhancing an individual's effort to become "more of a self." It also has great significance in contributing to the broader scale of human societal process. The theory additionally provides a conceptual framework for the exploration and integration of knowledge relevant to human behavior developing at all levels of the social and natural sciences. The exploration of knowledge developing in the sciences by individuals from a number of disciplines has been an important element in the ongoing development of Bowen theory since its first publication in 1966. Interestingly, the integration of scientific knowledge, I believe, enhances the effectiveness of one's clinical practice. The surface of our knowledge of the family and its influence on behavior has barely been scratched. It remains a wide-open field for those who decide to pursue it.

My initial interest in family systems was, like so many things in life, serendipitous. It occurred in the midst of an emergent and rapidly developing field described as "the family movement," taking place in the mental health field in the 1960s and 1970s. Beginning in the 1950s and 1960s at a number of sites around the country, the emergence of family research and therapy represented the beginning of a significant shift in thinking about human behavior. The research and clinical study of families led to the observation that individual behavior was highly regulated by the family. What had previously been understood to be a property of intrapsychic processes or personality characteristics was now seen by family researchers as interlinked with members of the relationship system of the family. To a young professional at that time, it was exciting to see this figure/ground shift in perspective taking place.

My first professional position was at a state mental hospital on a unit which housed patients who had been diagnosed with chronic schizophrenia. The twenty residents living on the unit had all been living in the state institution for more than twenty years. The position was a fortunate one for me as it entailed spending the full day on the unit, interacting with the patients. Though unsettling at first, after a short time, I became comfortable with psychotic behavior. As a result I came to know and care about them as individuals. With most of them it was possible for me to see beyond the symptoms they exhibited and see them as unique individuals, not just "schizophrenics." I was curious to learn more about their lives and the development of such profound disabilities.

The residents had been largely cut off from the outside world and few had any visitors or remaining contact with their families. My interest in learning more about them and their condition led me to read the "Progress Notes" in each patient's file. The almost daily notes had been entered over the twenty-plus years by hospital therapists, nurses, and psychiatrists. The notes contained descriptions about their initial hospitalizations and the symptoms they exhibited. They contained information about their social backgrounds and their initial diagnoses. Most were in their late teens or early twenties when hospitalized. The range of treatments they received over the years were also recorded, a number of which, though well-intentioned at the time, seemed cruel and depersonalizing.

It was clear in reading the notes of the various mental health professionals that most were interested in helping their patients. For the most part, the therapists' notes reflected their views that their help was resulting in slow but steady progress. It was clear that the professionals were invested in seeing their efforts as beneficial. They "saw" progress when in fact their patients were becoming increasingly institutionalized with no evidence of improvement.

As a young professional, I wondered how I might avoid falling into the same misguided belief in the effort to assist people, an effort which may simply be irrelevant or even contribute to their stasis. I wondered if there could be a way to be more objective about my efforts and not delude myself into thinking I was contributing to progress when I was not. I also wondered what might make a contribution to individuals exhibiting such problems. It was clear that the institutions and the various treatments they had been receiving had not.

I was also interested in the twofold effort of both gaining more self-knowledge and coming to see the world more "as it is" as opposed to seeing it through the lens of my developmental and cultural programming. It was a primary interest of mine and I believed it would also be an important element in my professional growth.

I was certainly not alone in my view that the institutionalization of individuals had deleterious effects on their lives. This was a period following the Mental Health Act of 1963 which resulted in a nationwide effort to keep the mentally ill in their communities and out of large institutions. This provided the context for my next two positions in the hospital, each of which led to my enduring interest in the family as central to the functioning and well-being of people. Following six months of working on the chronic patient unit, I took a position on what was called a crisis unit. The objective of the unit was to keep all new admissions to the hospital for less than two weeks. It involved an effort to stabilize the disturbed patient with medication and to keep the family involved during their stay. It was a remarkable experience for me.

I was able to witness how distraught the families were in hospitalizing one of their members. In meeting with the families, I learned of the behaviors and events which led to the point where they felt they could no longer keep the psychotic or suicidal family member at home. For the most part the family members were fearful and emotionally exhausted.

It was striking to see that the symptoms and behaviors of the newly admitted patients were similar to the ones I had read of those on the chronic unit when they were first hospitalized. It was rewarding to see that these newly hospitalized individuals would not spend their lives in an institution. Medication was often, but not always, helpful in stabilizing the highly disturbed patients. The engagement with their families during their stay also seemed to have a calming and stabilizing effect on them. For a number of the patients, however, this stabilization was short-lived after they returned home to live with their families. It was easy to come to the conclusion that these families negatively impacted their symptomatic member, leading to a readmission after several months or even weeks. Fortunately, my next position helped to expand my view on the part families played and led to my ongoing interest in family systems.

An interesting study designed to test the efficacy of avoiding hospitalizations of the mentally ill had been undertaken at Colorado State Hospital in the 1960s (Langsley & Kaplan, 1968). The study included 300 families seeking the hospitalization of a disturbed family member. The families were randomly assigned to a control group in which the member was admitted to the hospital and another to a group in which they were not hospitalized, but instead received brief family therapy in their homes. Follow-up studies (Langsley et al., 1968) at six and eighteen months later demonstrated that the families receiving family therapy in their homes had a lower recidivism rate than the hospitalized group, with one-sixth of the cost.

In 1969, a program based on this study was initiated at the state hospital in Chicago. I was invited to be a member of what was known as the Family Crisis Therapy team and fortunate to participate in the program for the following three years. It provided another outstanding learning experience for a young professional. Similar to the Colorado program, families seeking to hospitalize a member were told he or she would not be accepted at the hospital, but that a team of professionals would meet with them in their home that evening or the following day.

The program served three large communities in the inner city of Chicago, whose residents were primarily Hispanic, African American, or of Eastern European heritage. The objective of the program, in attempting to avoid a hospitalization, was to meet with families for six sessions and then to refer them to a community mental health center. The treatment team was fortunate to have two prominent family therapists as consultants. Dr. Robert MacGregor (1962) was involved in training the team in brief family therapy and as a weekly consultant, while Dr. Carl Whitaker (Neill & Kniskern,1982), who was then at the University of Wisconsin, consulted monthly at the hospital in family therapy.

The first family to be accepted into the program was memorable. It was on a Saturday evening and a young Puerto Rican family arrived at the hospital to have the father admitted. He was in his early thirties and accompanied by his wife and brother. In the previous couple of months, this man had become increasingly agitated and paranoid according to his family. The family had tried to calm him and convince him that his paranoid delusions were not founded in reality. The family feared for his safety and for those he had accused of trying to harm him. He had previously had a psychotic reaction and the family was visibly distressed.

After meeting with the family for an hour, they were told he would not be hospitalized, but that we would meet with the whole family at their home in the morning. They were asked to invite all of the concerned family members to be present. The family was apprehensive about this arrangement but seemed relieved that they would be attended to so quickly. It should be noted that medication was not prescribed at that point. The family and not the institution was given responsibility for this problem along with professional assistance in their home.

The next morning, a sunny Sunday, the crisis intervention team of three drove to the family address in the inner city. It was on a main street and we could not find a home at the address. A bar was open and we inquired about the address. The bartender responded that the family was in a back room of the bar and were waiting for us. On entering the room we discovered that more than twenty family members had assembled! Aunts, uncles, cousins, siblings, and in-laws were all there.

The meeting began by asking who would best be able to describe the concerns of the family about their member who had been so distressed. A brother was the primary spokesperson and described the behavior they had all become so alarmed about. A detailed history was gathered which included descriptions of this father's functioning prior to his break. Information was gathered about family events and significant changes which had occurred over the previous year. Hearing of the difficulties to which the family members had been responding to, broadened the context in which the psychotic reaction had occurred. Based on what was understood to be crisis intervention theory, only facts were sought with "who, what, when, and where" questions, while family comments that were more feeling-based were diverted. The father remained quiet and somewhat withdrawn throughout the meeting.

The meeting lasted for more than two hours. It was remarkable to observe the tension in the family slowly recede as they talked about the broader context of the family and its members. At times humorous comments were made. By the end of the meeting a plan was developed for the next meeting with just the immediate family. The family seemed relieved and appreciative and perhaps a bit more confident that they could manage this very difficult problem.

In this first meeting the context of the problem, as seen by the family, began to shift from the individual to a broader one. And the responsibility for addressing the problem and developing a plan shifted from the hospital to the family. The team's role was to be a resource to the family in their effort.

The team met with this family for six sessions. By the third meeting, the father no longer exhibited psychotic symptoms. This was by no means a cure, but the process clearly demonstrated that the father's psychotic reaction involved more than the father. A buildup of tension had been developing among family members over a prolonged period. This was evidenced by the reactions of multiple members to a number of stressful events and to one another. The family was not seen as the cause of the problem by the team, but it was evident that the reduction in family tension and fear which occurred over the course of the family therapy meetings alleviated the symptoms.

I was hooked. A novel and exciting new way of viewing human behavior was underway. This basic paradigmatic shift was occurring at a number of centers around the country. They all entailed a shift toward "systems thinking." I could intuitively grasp what systems thinking involved. I also knew that I had a very limited ability to think systems. But once a glimpse of it was stimulated by the observance of families, I knew it was something I wanted to acquire.

During the three-year period that I was a member of the Family Crisis Therapy team, I had the opportunity to meet with more than 200 families in their homes. A few were marital pairs isolated from their extended families, but the vast majority included nuclear family members with most involving extended families. Almost all the families were welcoming and invested in seeing if they could contribute to the recovery of the member who exhibited psychotic behavior or suicidal ideation.

I also attended countless seminars and conferences on family systems therapy during this period. I read the spectrum of new thinking emerging from various centers around the country and I continued to be enriched by the consultations with Carl Whitaker and Robert MacGregor. Despite my intellectual intoxication during this three-year period and the following three years at an outpatient mental health center, I grew frustrated with the slow progress I was making toward the goal of "systems thinking." I could "see" it in families, but I would lose it in the mid of a family's emotionality and the sense of urgency in wanting to help the families solve the myriad of very complex difficulties they were up against. I was attracted to a couple of family therapy approaches in particular, but for the most part those approaches were focused on the therapy, on techniques of family therapy. Each had conceptual frameworks underlying the therapy, which varied considerably. I found it was not possible to integrate the various frameworks due to the differences in their basic underlying orientations.

My frustration with my own slow development toward a goal of systems thinking, along with my difficulty in observing my own family with more clarity, led to the decision to seek a coherent conceptual framework. Carl Whitaker had emphasized the importance of the larger extended family and I could see its importance in the three- to four-generation families I had met with in the inner city of Chicago. My parents were immigrants, and I knew only those family members who had also immigrated to the United States. I knew little of those who had not emigrated or had emigrated to other countries.

I was also aware that my effectiveness as a family therapist would be related to how well I would come to know, understand, and function in my own family. After my initial six-year period in the field, I was frustrated with my slow pace in developing an ability to think systems with clinical families as well as the lack of progress I was making in relation to my own family. I decided that I needed to become grounded in one conceptual approach if I was to speed up my own learning. Of the various approaches, I chose to study the family systems theory which the family psychiatrist and researcher Murray Bowen had developed based on his research at the National Institute of Mental Health and later at Georgetown University. Though my knowledge of the theory was superficial at that time, the choice was based on two primary considerations: (1) the theory had a multigenerational perspective and (2) Bowen was the only investigator who had developed a process for working on self in one's own family. The choice to pursue knowledge of the family systems theory developed by Dr. Bowen was another fortunate development in my life.

My decision to attend the Georgetown Postgraduate Program in Family Systems Theory in 1975 was not serendipitous, but some of the consequences were. At that time the program, led by Dr. Bowen, was under the auspices of the Department of Psychiatry at Georgetown University Hospital in Washington, D.C. That same year it became a part of the newly formed Georgetown Family Center of which Murray Bowen was the director. I came away from the lectures by Dr. Bowen believing he was one of the finest systems thinkers I had yet encountered. I also came away with an understanding of the importance of theory, in the formal sense of the term, and the relevance of knowledge developing in the natural sciences. It opened up an expanded vista for the exploration of family, self, and human behavior. I was hooked once again by a new avenue for learning. My contact with Dr. Bowen continued until his death in 1990 and I continued to remain involved with the Georgetown Family Center (now known as The Bowen Center for the Study of the Family) to the present.

This book is about the family systems theory developed by Murray Bowen with an emphasis on the family as an emotional system and the development of a self. It is not a complete exposition of the theory. For those interested, I recommend the more basic texts (Bowen, 1978; Kerr & Bowen, 1988; Papero, 1990; Kerr, 2019). The theory has provided a rich framework for my exploration of human behavior, which includes the more than 2,000 clinical families I have had the privilege of seeing as well as my own family and self. It has also led me to explore a wide array of the scientific literature relevant to human behavior. In the course of developing a family systems theory, Murray Bowen also developed methods which can assist individuals and families in enhancing their capacity to effectively adapt to life's many challenges. The methods are based on the theory and require a grounding in Bowen theory. The emphasis in this approach is more on how a clinician or other individuals think about individual and family functioning than on methods of applying it. Acquiring the ability to "think systems" while relating to families and attaining a grounding in the theory and its application is a long-term, ongoing effort. While this book is focused on the theory and not so much on its application, I hope it may be one more resource for a person interested in this family systems theory and making gains in their own functioning, enhancing the ability to "think systems," and in contributing to the functioning of others.

I will cite some of the scientific literature which has expanded my interest and knowledge of individual and family behavior and which I believe has been both supportive of the theory and contributed to its development. The exploration of this literature, as well as contact with a number of remarkable scientists I cite, has not only enriched my knowledge but has been useful in making the theory my own. I hope that the presentation of my understanding of the theory will be of value to others and not distort in any way the theory itself. Each person has the capacity to explore the theory and to test it out for themselves in their own family, with clinical families, and/or with formal research. I believe this theory represents a major advancement in the knowledge of human behavior and that its application provides a pathway for enhancing the basic functioning of individuals and their families. I have taken the liberty to extensively use quotes from Dr. Bowen's original writings to capture some of his thinking and add some clarity to the discussion.

In *Family and Self*, I hope to capture Bowen theory's contribution to an understanding of the adaptive capacity of individuals and the role the family plays in it. Adaptive capacity can have several meanings and in chapter 1 I will present my view of its use in Bowen theory. I use the term "interchangeably" with the concept of differentiation of self, though the concept developed by Bowen is more refined. Differentiation of self is a rich concept, and the interested reader will need to further explore the concept in other available literature.

In the following chapters, I will present the contribution I believe Bowen theory makes to gain a more objective view of human behavior. Knowledge emerging in the neurosciences and in evolutionary biology are greatly contributing to a less subjective view of ourselves and our fellow humans, and Bowen theory, I believe, offers a way of integrating that knowledge. The theory also provides a framework for exploring the basic interdependence evident in the family and the role it plays in shaping our behavior and our relationships. Our remarkable brains give us the potential to observe ourselves and to become more objective about how we are influenced by our relationship systems and the part we each play in influencing them. This potential to be more objective can contribute to having more choice and as a result allow us to enhance the adaptive capacity of ourselves and our families.

Chapter 1

Family and Adaptive Capacity

The life of individuals can be said to begin with conception and end with death. In between, change is a constant throughout embryonic, neonatal, adolescent, and adult development. An orderly process is at play as cells grow and divide from the original zygote, as they differentiate to form tissues and organ systems. Development continues at birth as the newborn emerges from the protected environment of the mother's womb. Further changes are occurring as the infant grows and develops new capacities for self-regulation.

Completely helpless at birth, the newborn takes on, among others, the tasks of breathing, eating, and thermoregulation. Its immune, endocrine, and nervous systems rapidly develop to take on the challenges of living in this big new world. The process is astonishing in both its scope and complexity. From the third trimester through the second year of life, the brain is forming a million synapses a second. A million a second!

These changes and more are taking place throughout the prolonged period of human development, allowing individuals to adapt to their physical and social environments while maintaining a stable internal homeostasis. As social creatures, the relationship world is especially central to individuals in their effort to self-regulate and adapt to a changing environment. Development is not independent of the social context in which it occurs. The constant interchange infants and children experience, principally within the family, involves a reciprocal process taking place at both the physiological and psychological levels, shaping the very structure and functions of the brain (Branchi et al., 2013; Curley & Champagne, 2016; Fox et al., 2010; Lupien et al., 2009). Social interactions are now known to have a profound effect on our neural, endocrine, and immune systems as they respond to incoming signals from the social environment and trigger physiological and behavioral responses (Eisenberger & Cole, 2012; Szyf et al., 2008; Uvnas Moberg, 2003;

Walker et al., 2004). Psychologist John Cacioppo, one of the pioneers in the field known as social neuroscience, described this process well:

> the primary task of every organism in nature is to regulate itself in response to the environment. For social animals, a highly significant part of that environment is each other, and thus members of families, tribes, and villages regulate themselves as individuals while also influencing one another through what we have called co-regulation. The system of checks and balances involves physiology as well as behavior. (2008, p. 55)

In recent decades major advances have been made in understanding how the social environment shapes our very physiology. As Cacioppo noted, it is not a one-way process, but an interactive one from the beginning. Even prior to birth the embryo can regulate the mother's functioning through hormonal signaling, such as inducing her to increase her respiration, food intake, and level of available glucose (Champagne & Curley, 2015). The embryo in turn responds to maternal signaling (Szyf, 2019), which can also be influenced by the interactions between mother, father, and their social environment.

After birth, the growing awareness of the environment by the infant principally involves the social environment. By the age of three, following a remarkable period of brain growth, children begin a new level of self-regulation in relation to their world as they socially self-monitor in assessing how they fit in with the social group (Tomasello, 2019). The self-monitoring represents an active process occurring by all people in relationship systems as each member actively assesses how others are responding to them and they to others. This responsiveness, which is most obvious when we enter a new social setting, becomes more automatic and out of our awareness in our longstanding relationships. Throughout the course of an individual's life, social self-regulation is a central feature in adapting. Individuals differ in how well they self-regulate in relationship systems and the effort to understand such differences has engaged the work and thinking of investigators of many disciplines, from biologists to psychologists, from epidemiologists to sociologists, and from ethologists to anthropologists.

VARIATION AMONG INDIVIDUALS

Parents are generally amazed at how different each of their children is from their brothers or sisters. It is striking how the personalities, interests, and behaviors of siblings differ regardless of whether they are close in age, the same sex, or grow up in similarly stable or unstable family environments. The uniqueness of each child is easy to recognize. At the same time, it is interesting that while parents do not see strong similarities among their children, they often compare one or more as taking after one of the parents, grandparents, or another member of the extended family.

Many reasons are given in accounting for the differences and similarities among individuals such as genes or birth order. "She was born stubborn" or "He was always an easy-going child" can often be heard as parents describe a child. The birth order of children has been found to shape some differences in the personality characteristics of individuals. Frank Sulloway (1996) of MIT, for example, examined the birth orders of historically accomplished people in the arts, sciences, and politics to test his hypothesis that oldest siblings tend to identify with their parents and authority, thus being more likely to support the status quo. He posited that younger children are more likely to rebel against the established order. His hypotheses were generally supported as the accomplishments of first-borns were more likely to be conservative and supportive of the status quo, while those of later-borns were found to be more innovative or revolutionary.

Austrian psychologist Walter Toman (1961) found that based on their birth order and sex, sibling relationships influence their adult relationships. According to Toman, an older sister of a younger brother, for example, will likely differ in how she relates in her marital, parental, work, and other social relationships than a younger sister of an older brother. Dalton Conley (2004), a sociologist at New York University, found in his research that more than half of all income disparity occurs not between families, but within families. He cites a multitude of factors one of which he sees as the status hierarchy among siblings within the family. While other factors come in to play, early sibling relationships appear to account for some of the differences found among individuals.

Genetics obviously are a significant factor in accounting for individual differences among siblings, though an intermix of other factors have generally been found to be involved in accounting for the shaping of the adaptive capacity of individuals. There is evidence of a genetic influence on temperament and often such an influence can be seen early on. Harvard psychologist Jerome Kagan and others (Dilalla, Kagan, & Reznick, 1994), for example, found a genetic contribution to behavioral inhibition and uninhibition in children. Temperament in children by itself, however, has not been found to be a predictive factor related to their later life adaptiveness.

Researchers such as Thomas Boyce and Bruce Ellis (Boyce & Ellis, 2005; Ellis et al., 2011) have discussed another genetic factor influencing adaptive capacity: the influence of genes on the biological sensitivity some individuals have to their environment, heightening the degree to which they respond to beneficial or stressful early situations. There is evidence that the inheritance of some genetic polymorphisms, such as the serotonin transporter gene, can result in a child's heightened neuroendocrine stress reactivity to an adverse condition. Originally this was thought to be a vulnerability gene accounting for a range of emotional disorders. It has later been found that the biological sensitivity depended on context. The sensitivity to context might predispose an individual to negative health effects in an adverse environment, while at the same time have a beneficially adaptive effect in a more positive environment.

Both animal and human studies have clearly demonstrated the importance of early life experience in shaping the adaptive capacity of individuals in their adult life (Curley & Champagne, 2016; Dettmer & Suomi, 2014; Roth & Sweatt, 2011; Tang et al., 2006). Children who have experienced chronic stress have been found to be more vulnerable to both physical and emotional problems in their adult lives (Shonkoff et al., 2009; Szyf, 2019). The study of the hypothalamic-pituitary-adrenal (HPA) stress response system has demonstrated that the impact of stress during the prenatal and early postnatal periods have a more profound effect than during later development (Fox et al., 2010; Nusslock & Miller, 2016; O'Connor & Sefair, 2019). The impact of stressful events on an individual's adaptive capacity in adult life, however, does not appear to be a cause-and-effect relationship. Both the severity and duration of stressful events as well as a child's previous experience have also found to be factors (Essex et al., 2002: Lupien et al. 2009).

The observation that differences are found in the adaptive capacity of siblings growing up in the same family raises interesting questions which involve a number of factors. The same family can produce two siblings strikingly different in their life trajectories. As an adult, one sibling may have a stable family life, a successful career, and remain healthy into later life, while her brother flounders in all of these areas. In the effort to account for such differences, much of the literature has focused on characteristics inherent to an individual. In addition to their genetic makeup, personality type or early mother–child experience is frequently cited as determining one's basic adaptiveness in life. While genes may be one factor in successful or maladaptive adaptation, the nature/nurture dichotomy has in recent decades greatly receded as a greater intermix between genes and the environment has been discovered (Meaney, 2010).

At one time the influence of genes was thought to be unidirectional, an unfolding of a blueprint forming the individual phenotype from the inherited genotype. While this unfolding was occurring, the blueprint was viewed as influenced by the environment, but the genes themselves were thought to be untouched by the environment. More recently a revolution has occurred in our understanding of genetics as a host of an individual's genes have been found to either be expressed or silenced based on the relationship environment (Cole, 2013; Slavich & Cole, 2013; Young et al., 2019). In effect, the genome has been found to be more responsive to the environment than had previously been thought.

The parent–offspring relationship, in particular, has been discovered to influence brain development and behavior through epigenetic processes which increase or decrease gene expression without altering DNA sequences (Curley & Champagne, 2016; Meaney, 2010; Szyf et al., 2008). In describing the profound epigenetic impact the early parent–offspring relationship can have, Tie-Yuan Zhang and Michael Meaney (2010) write:

> There is now evidence that environmental events can directly modify the epigenetic state of the genome. Thus studies with rodent models suggest that during early development and in adult life, environmental signals can activate intracellular pathways that directly remodel the "epigenome," leading to changes in gene expression and neural function. These studies define a biological basis for the interplay between environmental signals and the genome in the regulation of individual differences in behavior, cognition, and physiology. (p. 438)

The environmental signals they are describing are occurring in the parent–offspring relationship. And epigenetic processes have been shown to be influential not just between a parent and child, but over several generations (Champagne, 2008). Frances Champagne and James Curley at the University of Texas describe the epigenetic process on parenting across the generations:

> Converging evidence from animal and human studies suggest that variation in or disruption to the quality of parent-offspring interactions can lead to divergent trajectories in brain development and behavior. These developmental effects may have far-reaching consequences that extend across generations. Though there are likely multiple pathways that contribute to these effects, epigenetic mechanisms have been proposed as a critical biological link between the experience of parenting and these within and across generation consequences. (Champagne & Curley, 2015 p. 73)

Variation in adaptive capacity has, of course, been central to natural selection and the diversity of species. From an evolutionary perspective, reproduction has generated variation in the adaptiveness of organisms in each generation over the course of life's 3.8-billion-year history on planet earth. Charles Darwin observed the range of variation existing within each species and recognized that each generation produces slight differences among offspring. He was fascinated by such differences and came to recognize that individual members of a species not only varied to a degree in their appearance but in the degree to which they successfully adapted to their environments. Darwin's observation of variation, and that not all individuals survived to reproduce, led to the development of the concept of natural selection, a process in which those characteristics enabling an organism to survive and reproduce are retained and carried into the future, while less adaptive characteristics are not. Over evolution's long history, slight variations occurring in the process of reproduction and their selection have led to the amazing variety of life on our planet.

The observation by Darwin that individuals of a species vary in degree represented a major shift in Western thought according to the evolutionary biologist Ernst Mayr (1982). It represented a shift from what Mayr termed "essentialistic thinking" to "population thinking." Essentialism, seen as dating back prior to Plato, has dominated Western thought. According to this perspective, all forms of life have a basic essence and all variations within a category are seen as deviations from this basic essence. It was argued that all triangles, for example, have a basic essence even though their forms may differ. A dog was viewed as having a basic essence shared by all dogs. The essence of a species, for example, was seen as eternal and not subject to change. This view, that all life forms have a basic essence, made it difficult to see the underlying continuity in life. Population thinking on the other hand views each individual as unique. Darwin's careful observation of many forms of life allowed him to see that all individual organisms simply varied in relation to one another. There is no essence, simply variation. It became clear to him that the offspring of sexually reproducing organisms were similar, but different. Essentialism is then seen more as a creation of the human mind than a fact of nature. This shift in thinking, from seeing individuals as expressions of unchanging essences to seeing each individual as unique, was central to the discovery of natural selection and evolution. Essentialist thinking remains prominent in today's world, however, and can be seen among the personality theories and diagnostic categories found in psychology and psychiatry.

The subject of this chapter is on the family influence on the development of the adaptive capacity of individuals and families, and in the variation found in this basic aspect of our lives. The conceptual framework attempting to account for these processes will be that of the family systems theory developed by the family psychiatrist and researcher Murray Bowen (1913–1990). In this theoretical perspective, the family is seen as an adaptive system in its own right, influencing all levels of complexity from genes to psychology to relationships. Within each family, variation among its members is generated in the process of family interactions occurring over the course of development. The resulting differences in adaptive capacity developing among individuals are quite stable throughout adult life. And the variation among siblings in each family can be observed to lead to a wider range of differences in basic adaptiveness over the future generations. While other factors contribute to differences among individuals, the family emotional system has been observed to entail basic nonrandom relationship patterns which predictably contribute to variation in basic adaptive capacity. The systems theory of the family, known as Bowen theory, represents a natural systems theory in which the family is viewed as a biopsychosocial system based on evolution. Bowen theory represents a significant departure from traditional theory in conceptualizing the functioning of individuals and families. In describing the development of his theory of the family, Bowen (2013b) wrote, "My concepts were framed in the orientation in the human as a biological-evolutionary creature" (p. 104). The integration of this orientation, systems thinking, and observation of the human family led to a new theory. The theory posits that the family is an adaptive system central to both individual development and variation among individuals in their basic adaptiveness.

ADAPTIVE CAPACITY

What is meant by adaptive capacity? In the broader context it refers to living systems at all levels of complexity in their ability to adjust to environmental threats or challenges and take advantage of its resources. From life's beginning, almost four billion years ago, all organisms encountered the ongoing challenge of survival. Molecular complexes formed, leading to the emergence of living cells separated from the environment by a membrane. The earliest unicellular forms of life required the capacity to maintain a stable internal integrity or homeostasis along with the ability to move toward and absorb nutrients in the environment along with avoiding toxins. In order for life forms to persist, reproduction was required. Life's history is one of persisting and reproducing. The replication of information contained in DNA base pair sequences (genes) was basic to heritability and the evolutionary process. In addition to survival and reproduction, the history of life has been one of simple forms evolving toward more complex ones. Single-celled microbes developed the capacity to adhere to one another and form larger complexes. When nutrients were rich, some microbes could operate as independent individuals. Under harsher conditions they could form colonies, increasing their capacity to adapt.

Bacteria evolved to form colonies of hundreds of thousands to millions. Though there is a cost to an individual bacterium in becoming part of a large cooperative colony, the advantages enhanced its ability to adapt to the environment. Bacterial colonies have been shown to have the capacity to process chemical signals which allow them to move toward nutrients and avoid toxins (Ben-Jacob et al., 2011). In contrast to life as an independent cell, the colony has the capacity to integrate more information from the environment, to store this information, and to respond more adaptively.

Slow for hundreds of millions of years, the pace of the evolution of complex forms of life began to increase with the emergence of nucleated cells
and later multicellular organisms (Libby & Rainey, 2013; Margulis, 1981;
Sapp, 2009). The first two billion years of life consisted of various forms of
cells called prokaryotes such as bacteria which lacked a nucleus. A significant
new development occurred in the evolution of life with the symbiotic merger
of what had previously been free-living unnucleated cells into larger cells
which now included a nucleus and other organelles. The larger nucleated or
eukaryotic cells represented the living together of different microbes each of
which had evolved to have different adaptive functions. The emergence of
this new level of complexity, which resulted from the fusion of once separate microbes, led to one of the great evolutionary transformations. As Lynn
Margulis, one of the early proponents of the symbiotic origin of nucleated
cells, and coauthor Dorian Sagan (2002) wrote, "The branches of the evolutionary tree fork, but they also fuse" (p. 202). Once the microbial merger
formed a nucleated cell about two billion years ago, it led to the emergence
of multicellular organisms with increasing capacities to adapt to the environment. The tree of life had greatly expanded in complexity and flourished.

The expansion of life forms resulted in the creation of countless new
econiches and new forms of adaptive capacity evolved. Our own species is a
product of this expansion. Following the divergence from our most common
primate ancestor over six million years ago, a remarkable evolution along the
hominin line occurred (Dunbar, 2016). The adaptive capacity of the members
of Homo sapiens can be seen as the result of these evolutionary experiments
leading to a species which has spread across this tiny planet. Appearing only
about 300,000 years ago, humans have demonstrated not only a remarkable
ability to adapt to a wide range of environments, they have also learned to
shape environments as they have adapted. This capacity, of course, is now
leading to the creation of an environment which will test the very adaptiveness of future generations of ours and other species (Wilson, 2012).

The use of the term "adaptiveness" can have several meanings which can
lead to some confusion. Adaptive can be used in the evolutionary sense and it
can also describe a phenotypic accommodation to an environmental change.
According to West-Eberhard (2003), when a change in behavior or physiology, due to phenotypic plasticity, occurs over the course of an individual's
development and contributes to the fitness or reproductive success of an individual, it can then be subject to natural selection. Following its spread through
a population, it can then be seen as adaptive in the evolutionary sense. I will
be using the term "adaptive capacity" to refer to the degree to which an individual or family is able to effectively respond to life challenges over lengthy
periods of time. Though genes, of course, contribute to adaptive capacity in
this sense, I am using the term to describe the functioning of individuals and

families and not in the ultimate (evolutionary) sense. I will be describing adaptive capacity as it is inferred from the concept of differentiation of self in Bowen theory. I would see differentiation of self as a phenotypic phenomenon as its variation among individuals and families is principally based on the multigenerational family emotional process. Changes in levels of differentiation are functional changes and do not require genomic change, though it is an open question as to the extent to which behavior might influence the genome in its expression or even its architecture (Cole, 2013; Meaney, 2010; Rubenstein et al., 2019).

With regard to humans, the subject of the adaptive capacity of individuals has been of interest to psychology for some time. In a review of concepts related to adaptive capacity, Frost (2020) describes some of the difficulties researchers have had in developing coherent conceptual frameworks. Concepts like resilience, coping, adaptation, and self-esteem all refer to traits or processes involving the capacity of individuals to respond effectively to threats or adversity, or their success in utilizing resources available to them. Variation among individuals in their adaptive capacity is described in the literature but a conceptual framework accounting for this variation in the larger human population has been limited.

In the broadest sense, the adaptive capacity of individuals can best be observed in their psychological, physiological, and social functioning over an extended period of years and during prolonged periods of stress. The context to which individuals must adapt, the length of time they are faced with significant stress, and how they respond at multiple levels must be taken into account. Variation in adaptive capacity can be observed when a number of individuals are subjected to the same stressful events or prolonged periods of adversity. Individuals experiencing identical stressors can vary in how the stressors are perceived and how effectively they respond to them (McEwen, 2007). Under prolonged, significant stress, the less adaptive individuals are more vulnerable to developing physical symptoms (i.e., cardiovascular, autoimmune, or gastrointestinal problems), emotional disorders (i.e., depression or disabling anxiety), or behavioral and relationship difficulties (i.e., domestic abuse). Individuals with greater adaptive capacity, in responding to the same stress, are more likely to effectively cope and evidence minimal or no symptoms. The prolonged and harsh conditions experienced by those attempting to escape life-threatening situations demonstrate both the amazing resilience of the human and a wide range in the capacity to adapt.

As Frost (2020) points out, most of the psychological literature on what more broadly can be described as adaptive capacity is based on an individual paradigm. Concepts such as resilience, coping, and adaptation generally refer to the capacity of the individual. Though context such as socioeconomic status or early life experience may be taken into account, the focus remains on

the individual. It has become increasingly obvious that the interactive reciprocal processes at play, within and between individuals, require a systems
conceptual framework integrating the multiple levels involved.

While much of psychiatry sought to establish various diagnostic categories
for the range of emotional disorders, Murray Bowen's study of human behavior led him to seek a way to place individual adaptiveness on a single continuum. Traditional psychiatry, for example, saw schizophrenia as a discrete
illness and different in kind from what had been seen as neurotic behavior.
Bowen saw individuals as varying in degree, but not in kind. His previous
work at the Menninger Foundation (1946–1954) in Topeka, Kansas, led him
to question some of the basic premises in psychiatry about schizophrenia
and other severe disorders (Kerr & Bowen, 1988). His study at the National
Institute of Mental Health (NIMH), beginning in 1954, allowed Bowen to
observe the differences as well as the underlying continuity at play among
family members.

The Family Study Project at NIMH (Bowen, 2013a) began with a focus
on mothers and their adult child diagnosed with schizophrenia. They lived
on the research unit and so could be observed daily by an around-the-clock
research and nursing staff. Two of the early observations in the study were
that the underlying interdependence between the mothers and their adult child
was more intense than had been expected and that the fathers were also a part
of the intense emotional process (Bowen, 2013a). Initially only the mothers
and their adult child lived on the research unit. Observations of the fathers,
who would visit on weekends, indicated that they had a significant effect on
the mother–child relationships. The fathers and siblings in the families were
then asked to reside on the unit. This led to the discovery that the families
functioned as a highly interdependent unit, with each member influencing
and being influenced by the others. The observed interdependence among
family members shed light on the degree to which they were not emotionally
separate but functioned as a unit. In an early paper Bowen (1960) described
the shift in observations which occurred during the research study:

> The schizophrenic psychosis of the patient is, in my opinion, a symptom mani-
> festation of an active process that involves the entire family. This orientation
> has evolved during the three and one-half years of a clinical research project in
> which schizophrenic patients and their parents have lived together on a psychi-
> atric ward in a research center. The family unit is regarded as a single organism
> and the patient is seen as that part of the family organism through which the
> overt symptoms of psychosis are expressed. (Reprinted in Bowen, 1978, p. 45)

Other less symptomatic families were seen on an outpatient basis during
this period and though less exaggerated, the same basic relationship patterns

were observed. The fact that these patterns were more exaggerated in the families with schizophrenia than in the less symptomatic families contributed to the discovery that the same basic family patterns could be observed in all families.

DIFFERENTIATION OF SELF

Early on in his investigations, Bowen searched for a way to conceptualize basic differences among people in their functioning or adaptiveness. He observed that people varied in their degree of maturity (Bowen, 2013a; Butler, 2015). The parents of the schizophrenic patients were observed to be more mature than their symptomatic son or daughter, but only in degree. Likewise, the less symptomatic outpatient families were seen as more mature, but again only in degree.

While the interdependence among family members could be observed, there was variation in their degree of dependence. Bowen described the parents and adult child with schizophrenia functioning as "a three-legged stool." The other siblings, though a part of the family unit, were less emotionally dependent on the parents and less vulnerable to being drawn into the emotional process. The parents were observed to be equally immature. In a paper shortly after the research study ended, Bowen wrote,

> There is an intense interdependence between father, mother, and patient which we have called the "interdependent triad." It is usual for normal siblings to become rather involved in the family problem, but not so deeply that they cannot separate themselves from the triad, leaving the father, mother and patient interlocked in the family oneness. (Bowen, 2013a, p. 111)

The difficulty in separating or remaining locked into a "family oneness" represented one end on a continuum of maturation. The failure of a child to separate from the parental family was observed to result in a constraint on development and in their capacity to adapt in adult life. Schizophrenia is one example, but the lack in the development of adaptive capacity can be found in other examples of individuals unable to move into adult functioning. At the low end of a continuum of maturity, individuals can be seen as principally regulated by the relationship environment with little capacity for self-regulation or the development of a self. Chronic alcohol or drug addiction and criminality are other manifestations of immaturity or emotional dependence. At an extreme level of dependency, individuals may be unable to live apart from the family or institutions. Another expression of heightened dependence on family can be found among those who have great difficulty in tolerating social interactions and so isolate themselves to avoid the inherent tension they experience in close relationships (Kerr, 2019).

Bowen also sought to identify those people who would represent the other end of a continuum, those who function at high levels in most areas of their lives. What did those individuals look like and what are the characteristics that could indicate where on a continuum of adaptiveness or maturity all individuals could be placed?

The observation of variation in levels of maturity among individuals led to the development of the formal concept of differentiation of self (Bowen, 1978). In the effort to move toward science, Bowen sought to use terms that were consistent with biology and the natural sciences. He used the term "differentiation" analogously to the process in which cells differentiate from one another. In the family, offspring could be observed to emotionally separate from the parental family but only to a degree. "Emotional oneness" could be observed in all families, though greater in some than others. Over the course of development, individuals move toward increasing levels of emotional autonomy, but some degree of what Bowen described as "unresolved emotional attachment" or dependence remains on reaching adulthood. The level of unresolved emotional attachment is seen as related to the degree of maturity, or lack of it, an individual attains over the course of development.

Bowen searched for indicators of variation among individuals in the levels of maturity or differentiation they attained. This led to the observation that individuals differ in the degree to which they are able to distinguish between their feelings and their thinking. He developed a continuum or scale of differentiation based on this characteristic. Bowen (1978) wrote:

> The core of my theory has to do with the degree to which people are able to distinguish between the *feeling* process and the *intellectual* process. Early in the research, we found that the parents of schizophrenic people, who appear on the surface to function well, have difficulty distinguishing between the subjective feeling process and the more objective thinking process. This is most marked in a close relationship. This led to investigation of the same phenomenon in all levels of families from the most impaired, to normal, to the highest functioning people we could find. We found that there are differences between the ways feelings and intellect are either fused or differentiated from each other, and this led us to develop the concept of differentiation of self. (p. 355)

It is a rich concept with many dimensions and will not be adequately covered in this book. A fuller description of the concept is found in Bowen's own writings (Bowen, 1978) and Kerr (2019). One of the difficulties many people have in grasping the meaning of this concept is in viewing it from what might be described as an individual paradigm. The development of the family systems theory by Bowen represented a shift to a new paradigm, one that might be called a "natural systems paradigm," differing significantly from the predominant paradigm of individualism. In describing a fundamental shift beginning to occur in biology, based on the development of new instruments, Gilbert, Sapp, and Tauber (2012) write,

These discoveries have profoundly challenged the generally accepted view of "individuals." Symbiosis is becoming a core principle of contemporary biology, and it is replacing an essentialist conception of "individuality" with a conception congruent with the larger systems approach now pushing the life sciences in diverse directions. (p. 326)

Bowen's theory of the family represented such a development. For much of the twentieth century, the predominant paradigm in psychiatry was that of Freud's psychoanalytic theory and its many variants. In later decades, the view shifted to one in which the more severe disorders were seen as based on brain chemistry and structure (Bentall, 2004). The focus in psychiatry has remained largely based on an individual paradigm. When viewed from an individual perspective or paradigm, psychiatric disorders are viewed as personality characteristics or neurological defects emanating from the intrapsychic or neural processes of the individual. Disorders may be seen to be influenced by the parent–child relationship or other environmental factors during development, but they are viewed as an individual characteristic. In the strict sense of the term introduced by Thomas Kuhn (2012), the shift to a new paradigm in thinking creates obstacles for those whose way of thinking remains embedded in the previous paradigm. The concept of differentiation of self is a systems concept based on relationship processes. Locating the source of behavior in the individual and as separate from relationship processes generally leads to what can be called "cause and effect" or "linear thinking" which differs substantially from systems thinking (Kerr, 2019).

Another misperception of differentiation of self is that it is a psychological concept. In developing the concept, Bowen saw it as based on biology. It entails psychological and social processes but is posited to be deeply rooted in the very biology and evolution of Homo sapiens. A clearer view of the biological and evolutionary basis of the concept can be appreciated through knowledge of the evolution of the nervous system and the brain. While the concept of the emotional system as defined in Bowen theory is viewed as extending to life's earliest beginnings, the evolution of the nervous system and brain portrays a movement toward an increasing capacity for the regulation of an organism's internal milieu and flexibility in responding to its environment. The human capacity to respond thoughtfully to life's many challenges is an outgrowth of this process and the concept of differentiation of self reflects the degree to which this capacity varies among people.

Differentiation of self is central to Bowen theory, but it is one of eight inter-related concepts which will be presented later in this book. As a systems theory, each concept is related to the others, each referring to processes at play in the family. An individual's level of differentiation of self, for example, must necessarily be considered in the context of the nuclear family emotional process and the multigenerational family process (Bowen, 1978; Noone, 2015).

Bowen described that the development of his family systems theory occurred rapidly during the six-year period between 1957 and 1963. First published in 1966, the theory was based on his experience and research at Menninger and NIMH. Seeking to move toward a science of human behavior he wrote,

> In those years, I was strongly influenced by readings and lectures in aspects of evolution, biology, the balance of nature, and the natural sciences. I was trying to view man as a part of nature rather than separate from nature. (Bowen, 1978 p. 359)

As mentioned earlier, by the early 1960s he came to see that all levels of human functioning could be seen to exist on a continuum, which he initially described as a "scale of differentiation of self" (Bowen, 1978 p. 161). This marked a significant change in the conceptualization of human behavior. The concept can be understood as a continuum of variation in the degree to which people mature on reaching young adulthood. A highly refined formulation of what is entailed in "maturity," differentiation of self is a broad concept entailing the development and functioning of individuals within the context of the family relationship system. It cannot be understood apart from what Bowen defined as the emotional system.

The family emotional system, as defined by Bowen, will be presented in more detail in chapter 4, but it can briefly be described as an adaptive system, a biopsychosocial system based on evolution. The family is often seen as a social or cultural phenomenon, but in defining it as an emotional system, Bowen theory refers to its biological basis. Seen as a natural system, the family is squarely placed in its evolutionary context, subject to the laws influencing all living systems. Culture may influence how family process is expressed, but the basic family emotional process is seen as universal. It is important to note again that Bowen theory, in positing that the family emotional system is a product of evolution, does not attempt to define how the family evolved but how it functions.

The concept of differentiation of self is a developmental concept as well as a concept referring to the basic adaptiveness of people throughout their life course. As a developmental concept it refers to a process occurring from the prenatal period through late adolescence or young adulthood. Individuals move from a state of complete dependence in utero toward attaining increasing levels of regulating self of increasing autonomy. The movement toward emotional autonomy and an increasing capacity to manage life's myriad challenges occurs in the context of the family. Having the potential to both enhance and constrain the maturational process, family is viewed as central to a person's growth and development, resulting for individuals in a balance of self-regulating and other-regulating processes.

Over the course of development, the differentiation of the higher cortical systems, or what Bowen defined as the intellectual system, is seen as involving the degree to which they can be utilized by individuals in responding to life challenges. When these systems are less well-developed or differentiated, the more automatic emotional processes have more influence in determining behavior. The range between these two extremes will reflect a continuum in adaptive capacity or differentiation of self. This will be more fully discussed in chapter 3.

The maturational process of an individual's separating out from the family is often heard as emotionally distancing rather than the development of a separate self in the family system. Differentiation of self corresponds to the level of maturity attained over the course of development. According to Bowen theory, the greater the maturity of an individual, the more capacity he or she has to relate more freely and openly with one's family and in other important relationships. At greater levels of maturity, the thoughts, feelings, and behaviors of individuals are less constrained or determined by the relationship system.

The constraints on emotional autonomy or differentiation of self are based on a family's multigenerational history, played out in the interactional processes observable in the present. In Bowen theory, the human family is seen as a self-regulating system, maintaining an ongoing homeostasis over time. The homeostasis results from the interactions and functioning of its members as they seek to adapt to one another and the larger environmental context. It represents a process involving both the effort to regulate the others to whom we are attached and to comply with or resist the efforts of the others to regulate ourselves. Each individual then operates in an ongoing process of self-regulation and other-regulation or what Bowen described as a balance of individuality and togetherness. It is in this exquisite interchange, occurring largely out of awareness, that development takes place. More basic than feelings, the emotional processes involved in maintaining a stable internal homeostasis while adapting to the environment, were seen by Bowen as basic to all of life. The emotional system as conceived by Bowen underpins the adaptive behavior of living systems, extending back through the eons of evolution.

The concept of differentiation of self refers to the adaptive capacity of individuals, though it has a more defined meaning and entails more elements. The assessment of an individual's level of differentiation of self requires knowledge of his or her functioning over a span of time involving periods of both more and less stress. It also requires knowledge of how that individual functions in the family as well as how the family has been functioning during those periods. As will be discussed in chapter 4, the better functioning of one family member may be dependent on the lesser functioning of a spouse or child. The basic level of differentiation of self among members of a nuclear family unit may vary, but the differences are not widespread. The functioning of individuals in a family may be significantly different and may vary over time, but this generally refers to what is described as functional levels of differentiation rather than basic levels (Bowen, 1978; Kerr, 2019). Functional levels of differentiation vary with changes in the conditions of an individual's life, while basic levels are observed to be more stable through good and bad times. Siblings may emerge from their family at different basic levels of differentiation of self, but they remain in the same ballpark as that of their parents.

A not uncommon example of differences in functional levels of differentiation in a family can be observed in a marriage in which one spouse may function at a pretty good level—free from symptoms and performing well in his or her career—while the other may function poorly with psychiatric, physical, or behavioral symptoms. From a systems perspective, this can be observed as a reciprocal process with an underlying dependency at play, a process in which the functioning of each is based on the functioning of the other. A consistent observation is that individuals select a life partner at similar levels of maturity or differentiation of self, even though over the course of a marriage their functioning may develop into a reciprocal pattern in which one functions at a more adequate level, while the other appears less adaptive. The underlying emotional dependence or maturity of each is seen as remaining similar.

Another important variable to be taken into account in distinguishing between an individual's basic versus functional level of differentiation of self is that of chronic anxiety. While one's basic level of differentiation is seen as quite stable throughout adulthood, the functional level can vary more widely depending on the level of one's chronic anxiety. For the most part, an individual's level of chronic anxiety is related to one's level of differentiation. At higher levels of differentiation, the chronic anxiety of individuals is less than those at lower levels. This again reflects adaptive capacity, the capacity to accurately assess and respond to life's challenges. Anxiety is basic to all of life and is a vital element in assisting an organism to be on the lookout for potential threats and in mobilizing responses to them. Bowen theory posits that those individuals at higher levels of differentiation can more accurately read real or potential threats, while those at lower levels will be more vulnerable to either overrespond or under-respond to perceived threats.

A principal factor contributing to one's level of chronic anxiety is the degree of dependence one has on others for their functioning. In describing the association between adaptive capacity and chronic anxiety, Kerr (1992) writes,

> Level of adaptiveness roughly correlates with level of chronic anxiety. Given sufficiently adverse circumstances, anyone can experience periods of heightened chronic anxiety, but poorly adaptive people tend to have more chronic anxiety than those who are more adaptive. The correlation between chronic anxiety and adaptiveness stems, to a significant extent, from the fact that the least adaptive people are the most heavily dependent on others for their emotional well-being. Preoccupation with being loved, accepted, and approved of, and with being able to manage one's own life effectively, although characteristic of all people to some degree, reaches an extreme at the least adaptive end of the continuum. Dependence on the opinions and actions of others and uncertainty about decision making breed chronic anxiety. (1992, pp. 101–102)

It is quite a leap from a position of observing behavior at the level of the individual or seeing the family as a collection of individual personalities to one of observing the family as a unit and provides a different view of the adaptive capacity of individuals. The shift to an observational lens focused on the level of the family unit provided Bowen with a wealth of observations which had not previously been available. It permitted a different view of what underlies human behavior. If the observation that the family functions as a self-regulating system, as a unit, is accurate, it provides a conceptual framework for observing behavior with markedly less subjectivity. Bowen's conceptualization of the family as an emotional system also provided a framework for the integration of knowledge developing in the sciences across many disciplines. As Daniel Papero (2015) writes,

> This broad conceptual framework (Bowen theory), a natural systems framework of the human, permits the incorporation of findings from many areas of biological science and may allow the development of an integrated theory of the human, one that links the biochemistry of cellular interaction to the behavioral reciprocity of relationship interaction. (p. 28)

In his book *Behave: The Biology of Humans at Our Best and Worst*, biologist Robert Sapolsky (2017) presents a wide range of current knowledge regarding many of the variables influencing human behavior. He discusses such variables as genetic makeup, development, neurobiology, and more in describing a number of the levels of complexity involved in an individual's behavior. In the effort to account for the range of behavior from our "worst to our best," he covers many of the areas that go into determining an individual's adaptive capacity. The various levels he describes involve complex, interactive systems. What is missing is a systems theory or conceptual framework allowing for the integration of the biological, psychological, and social processes involved in behavior, one which attempts to account for the variation in adaptiveness among individuals.

The concept of differentiation of self and the systems theory of the family developed by Bowen represents such an effort. The future will determine whether this theory will prove to be a productive one contributing to a science of human behavior. It is my view that knowledge about the family and how its functioning contributes to the range of adaptive capacity of individuals will necessarily be included in a science of human behavior. Obviously much remains unknown. The term "self" itself is difficult to pin down and must be dealt with at the theoretical level. For some, self is a property of consciousness and is based on self-awareness. Others see self as more basic and as involving much more. Neuroscientist Joseph LeDoux (2002) writes, "The existence of a self is a fundamental concomitant of being an animal. All animals, in other words, have a self, regardless of whether they have the capacity for self-awareness" (p. 27). He later describes an aspect of self which resonates with its use in Bowen theory:

> The machinery (of self) includes all of the biological requirements of being a self-sustaining organism, including a set of mutually compatible genes, immunological self-recognition, and a homeostatic mechanism that maintains self-regulating body functions. It also includes a variety of behavioral tendencies, often referred to as personality or temperament, that depend on either genetic influences or learning and that are expressed automatically—you don't have to consciously remember your core personality. (LeDoux, 2019 p. 297)

Bowen (1988) had previously defined self in a similarly broad manner in writing:

> The "self" is composed of constitutional, physical, physiological, biological, genetic and cellular reactivity factors as they move in unison with psychological factors. On a simple level, it is composed of the confluence of more fixed personality factors as they move in unison with rapidly moving psychological states. Each factor influences the other and is influenced by the others. (p. 342)

A number of neuroscientists see self as including more than the interior of the individual and involving aspects of an individual's environment over the course of development and in the present. Bowen theory describes the developmental process of the differentiation or maturation of self from the family "oneness." This includes the differentiation of the higher cortical systems involved in what Bowen defined as the intellectual system. It is in the family emotional system that this process occurs, shaping differences in the adaptive capacity of individuals.

In summary the maturation or differentiation of self, according to Bowen theory, entails two interrelated and basic processes: (1) the development of emotional autonomy in relation to an individual's family of origin and (2) the differentiation in the functioning of higher cortical systems (intellectual system) involved in effective self-regulation.

In the following chapters, I will discuss some of the central concepts of Bowen theory, concepts based on observations of the family with an objective of understanding some of the variables influencing differences in the adaptive capacity of individuals and families. Despite the amazing amount of knowledge that has been discovered about human behavior, it is obvious that the surface remains only scratched.

Chapter 2

Toward Emotional Objectivity

The idea of "emotional objectivity" can provide for endless discussion and debate. For many, placing the two words together seems odd and represents opposite poles. Our elaborate brains allow for the observation and processing of simple to very complex aspects of the world beyond our skin. For the most part we go through each day with the assumption that we are seeing the world "as it is." And this impression is continuously reinforced by our daily experiences.

Our experience, however, is being processed through our moist three-pound brain and nervous system. And the processing of our experience is greatly colored by our previous experience as well as by the context in which it occurs (Kahneman, 2011). The debate about how accurately we are able to perceive the world and ourselves goes back to pre-Socratic times and continues into the present. Is there a natural world that exists independently of the human mind? Most of those engaged in the scientific endeavor would fall on the side of saying yes. Is it possible for the human to come to know the natural world "as it exists"? Again, most scientists would probably respond affirmatively, but acknowledge the limitations in attaining complete knowledge. The limitations include not only how much remains unknown but the degree to which our inherent subjectivity and observational blindness prevent us from truly seeing the world "as it is." Will the human be able to develop a science of human behavior? Is it possible to become objective about ourselves and our species? My guess is that the response to these questions among scientists will vary more. Our observational blindness and the degree of our subjectivity become more apparent the closer we get to the study of ourselves. It would seem it is difficult for most to recognize that we are not the independent beings that our subjectivity might lead us to believe. If it is difficult to truly see ourselves as interdependently linked to all of life, the recognition that we occupy functional positions in our families and that our thoughts, feelings, and behaviors are significantly based on our interdependent family relationships is especially difficult. As Michael Kerr writes,

> If the family is an emotional unit, then people often function in ways that are a reflection of what is occurring around them. They have precious little autonomy from their environment. The thoughts, feelings, and behavior of each family member, in other words, both contribute to *and* reflect what is occurring in the family as a whole. (Kerr & Bowen, 1988 p. 9)

Contributing to this "blindness" are the many underlying and unspoken assumptions we make about ourselves and the world around us. The history of science is replete with assumptions or perspectives about the world that served to obstruct viewing phenomena in nature which existed in front of our very eyes. Many of the assumptions or communal mindsets serving as obstacles were remnants from the past and views and beliefs constructed in the effort to make sense of the natural world and our place in it. The world's great religions all provide such explanations, but they are also found in the histories of philosophy and science.

In 1912, for example, the Austrian Alfred Wegener suggested that at one point in the planet's history, the various continents had formed one large continent. He noticed that the shape of the present continents seemed to fit together like a jigsaw puzzle and that they may have drifted apart over millions of years. His hypothesis of "continental drift" was ridiculed by geologists. Over the years, however, evidence continued to mount that his hypothesis was accurate. It wasn't until the 1960s that "plate tectonics" was accepted as a fact.

Despite the limitations of our subjectivity, curiosity about the natural world has also been an intrinsic characteristic of our species. Curiosity and an interest in making sense of life and the world have been evident among humans for millennia. The emergence of science, a relatively recent development in Homo sapiens' brief history, has provided a process for moving toward a less subjective or more objective view of the world. The early beginnings of science can be found among the philosophers and physicians of ancient Greece. Religion and philosophy dominated explanatory efforts during the Middle Ages and the Renaissance. Despite strong initial resistance in their societies, the observations of Copernicus and Galileo greatly contributed to a more objective view of planetary movements. While their discoveries overturned entrenched views of the centrality of the human's place in the cosmos, their observations were of phenomena far removed from life on planet earth. It was not until the middle of the eighteenth century that biology began to more clearly separate itself out from religion and philosophy (Mayr, 1982).

The Israeli historian Yuval Harari (2015) posits that a principal factor driving the emergence of science in the Western world was the growing awareness that we did not know the answers to many of the questions raised about the natural world. He writes:

> The Scientific Revolution has not been a revolution of knowledge. It has been above all a revolution of ignorance. The great discovery that launched the Scientific Revolution was the discovery that humans did not know the answers to their most important questions.

> Modern day science is a unique tradition of knowledge, inasmuch as it openly admits *collective* ignorance regarding *the most important questions*. (2015, p. 251–52)

Given the limitations of the subjective mind, it is not surprising that the effort to move toward objectivity has been more difficult the closer it has come to viewing ourselves. The discovery of planetary movements and the place of our own planet in the solar system were highly disturbing, though of distant phenomena. Darwin's discovery contributed to the erosion of a subjective view of ourselves and the world in which we live, placing us within the context of an evolved form of life and not separate from the natural world. But for the most part psychology and psychiatry largely ignored Darwin and evolution until the end of the twentieth century.

Sigmund Freud was interested in science and hoped to develop a scientific theory of human behavior. His observations, that much of human behavior was instinctual and occurred outside of an individual's awareness, was a radical departure from the accepted views of the time. He also observed how much adult behavior was shaped by the early parental relations, especially with mother. His theory became foundational for psychiatry and much of psychology in the first half of the twentieth century. He developed a form of psychotherapy which continues to the present. Psychoanalytic theory, though often unknowingly, has also continued to be influential in a good many of the current approaches which are based on what can be described as the centrality of the "therapeutic relationship."

By the middle of the last century, an increasing criticism of psychoanalysis emerged that it was not scientific. In psychiatry a paradigm shift began to occur with the promise of psychotropic medications for the more severe forms of emotional disorders. This led to a view that such disorders had a biological basis and psychiatry moved rapidly in the direction of treating emotional disorders as neurological defects or chemical imbalances in the brain (Bentall, 2009). The neuroscientist and Nobel Prize winner Eric Kandel's book *In Search of Memory: The Emergence of a New Science of*

Mind vividly captures some of the transformations which were occurring in psychiatry. This paradigmatic shift toward "a new science of the mind" was influenced by knowledge developing in the neurosciences, which went beyond a focus on pathology to broader areas of human behavior (Gazzaniga, 1992). The advances in neuroscience over the past half century have been astonishing and have certainly contributed to the effort to move toward a science of human behavior.

Another effort to become more scientific was represented by the development of behaviorism which was dominant in psychology for the first half of the twentieth century. Behaviorism attempted to deal with subjectivity by eliminating the study of all phenomena between a stimulus and the behavioral response to it. It represented an effort to include only observable facts and treated all that occurred between a stimulus and a response as a "black box." The effect of this approach was a cause and effect or linear view of behavior and as a result had difficulty in accounting for complex interactive processes. Evolutionary thinking was largely seen as unnecessary.

Psychoanalytic theory did include the study of feelings and emotions, but despite its prevalence in psychiatry, the study of this central feature of human behavior was largely avoided for decades. As Antonio Damasio (1999) writes,

> By the end of the nineteenth century Charles Darwin, William James, and Sigmund Freud had written extensively on different aspects of emotion and given emotion a privileged place in scientific discourse. Yet, throughout the twentieth century and until quite recently, both neuroscience and cognitive science gave emotion a very cold shoulder. (p. 38)

To some degree most of the conceptual approaches in psychology and the field of mental health have been concerned with the adaptive capacity of individuals. Whether the focus has been on the development and classification of psychiatric symptoms and difficulties in adapting (Bentall, 2004) or on defining what might be optimal for the human (Maslow, 1971), an understanding of the full range of behavior has been the subject of study. The effort to understand human behavior from a scientific perspective has involved, directly or indirectly, almost all of the life and social sciences. In recent decades the neurosciences can be said to have gained ascendancy. Some of the knowledge developing in the neurosciences which shed light on the adaptive capacity of individuals will be discussed in the next two chapters.

Murray Bowen was among those in psychiatry in the middle of the last century who began to question whether psychoanalysis, the predominant theory at the time, could become scientific. He initially became grounded in psychoanalytic theory with a goal of contributing to it becoming more scientific. Initially, discrepancies arose for him between the theory and his clinical observations. Though it was unorthodox at the time to see family members of patients who were in psychotherapy, Bowen was intrigued by the impact family members had on the functioning of patients and began to meet with some of them when they visited the clinic. It was not long before he began to believe that some of this theory's underlying assumptions and concepts presented obstacles to a move toward science. He wrote,

> Psychoanalytic theory was formulated from a detailed study of the individual patient. Concepts about the family were derived more from the patient's perceptions than from direct observation of the family. From this theoretical position, the focus was on the patient and the family was outside the immediate field of theoretical and therapeutic interest. Individual theory was built on a medical model with its concepts of etiology, the diagnosis of pathology in the patient, and treatment of sickness in the individual. Also inherent in the model are the subtle implications that the patient is the helpless victim of a disease or malevolent forces outside his control. A conceptual dilemma was posed when the most important person in a patient's life was considered to be the cause of his illness, and pathogenic to him. (Bowen 1978, p. 148)

Murray Bowen was an astute observer of human behavior. As mentioned earlier, the shift to observing the family as an emotional unit occurred during his research at National Institute of Mental Health (NIMH). But this observation was the result of years of observing, study, and seeking a way to move toward a science of human behavior. It resulted in a view of the family as a natural system regulated by processes at play in all of life on earth. Central to his effort to observe human behavior "as it is" was an objective to be aware of the degree to which subjectivity determines what is seen and to focus on what Bowen described as "functional facts" (Bowen, 1978). An underlying premise in Bowen's research, that the human family exists independently of what the human thinks it is, captures his effort to move toward science and toward a less subjective or more objective view of human behavior. He wrote,

> The focus on the family instead of the individual provided a completely different thinking dimension. The previous years of study may have figured into entire families living on the (research) ward together. The study played a monumental part in the research itself and in the subsequent twenty-five years. With the families living together, I could *see* a completely different world. Years of work suddenly became clear. The view faded in and out until I could control it better. It was there when I could think about evolution and science. (Bowen, 2013b p. 103)

The observation that the family functioned as a unit led to a new level in the study of behavior. The move from the study of intrapsychic processes to mother–child dyads to the family unit allowed for the observation of repeated interactional patterns of behavior which could be observed and recorded. It represented a shift analogous to the one made by Stanford biologist Deborah Gordon in her study of harvester ants. Her study led to the observation that the ant colonies functioned as complex adaptive systems. The study of individual ants alone did not allow for the observation of how their behavior functioned as components in the larger colony and how the colony regulated the behavior of the individual ants. She writes,

> over the last 15 years, it has become clear that many biological systems are regulated by networks of interaction among the components, from genes to individuals. It is colonies, not individuals, that behave in a predictable way. (Gordon, 2010, p. 46)

The shift in the observational lens from the individual to the family unit led Bowen and the research team at the NIMH Family Studies Project to a similar discovery. A change in one family member or relationship could be seen to result in change in another. Tracking interactional behaviors of family members resulted in the observation of stable relationship patterns which could be observed in the research families (Bowen, 2013a). The study of outpatient families found similar patterns, though less exaggerated. The research focused on what people did and not on what they said. A disciplined effort centered on "how, what, when and where" questions rather than "why" questions. What emerged was a form of systems thinking that sought to observe what Bowen described as the "functional facts" occurring in the relationship interactions. A functional fact would be a predictable change in emotional functioning of one family member in response to a predictable social cue in another (Kerr 2019, p. 90).

An example of functional facts is represented in a relationship pattern between two spouses. Their relationship had become increasingly distant and conflictual over several years. The wife saw her husband as controlling and demanding, while the husband saw his wife as distant and cold. Each saw the other as the problem and each became more frustrated as the emotional intensity in their relationship became more exaggerated. In a sense each felt they were the victim of the other. The husband said his only expectations were that he be loved by her and receive affection from his wife. Sex and intimacy were absent in their relationship and he blamed his frustration on her withholding behavior. The wife saw her husband as lacking respect for her in demanding not only more affection but that she agrees with his views on money matters and parenting.

Some of the functional facts in the relationship were that when he pressured his wife to be more affectionate, she would become more emotionally distant. Likewise, as she became more distant, he saw her as being "unloving." The functional facts consisted of the predictable behaviors resulting from their subjective feeling states. Once they could begin to observe how their own behavior contributed to a relationship pattern, the level of blaming began to decrease. They began to see themselves less as victims of the other. The husband began to see that his own emotional dependence on his wife could be "suffocating" to her. He could begin to recognize the impact of his pressure on his wife to solve his emotional dependency was having on her. The wife began to see how her distancing or "shrinking" in response to his efforts to have her comply with his demands for affection as well as in matters of finance and parenting represented a lack of defining her own functioning in the relationship. Rather than view him as controlling, she became clearer about gaining more control over her own behavior and developing her own positions on matters important to her.

The functional facts in this example involve the predictable behaviors each one demonstrates in response to the behaviors and feeling states of the other. From this perspective, neither is "causing" the response of the other, but each is participating in an observable process or pattern. It is unnecessary to understand "why" one is feeling rejected when such reciprocal processes can be observed. And when one person can observe their part and begin to take responsibility to their contribution in the process, the pattern and behaviors involved will be modified. As Kerr (2019) writes, "The term *functioning position* refers to how a person's position in a relationship system regulates that person's functioning and contributes to a system process" (p. 91).

The step back from observing the individual to observing the unit opened a significantly new dimension and a way of dealing with the influence of subjectivity in the study of human behavior. Similar to Gordon's study of ant colonies, the family can be seen as behaving more predictably than its individual members. The family unit is observable. It does not require interpretations regarding the internal motivations for the behavior of individuals any more than it would for chimpanzees in a troop or ants in a colony. The family was observed to evidence predictable behavioral patterns which can be observed and recorded. Individual behaviors could now be seen as functional components of the family unit, revealing patterns of behavior not previously observed.

Our subjectivity is evident in the difficulty we have in truly grasping the degree to which our individual selves are interdependently embedded in the present and with the past. Far from being the autonomous, free-willed individuals our subjective experience can lead us to believe we are, the facts of life indicate our lives and our behavior are shaped by countless interacting elements. Our lives are rooted not only in our evolutionary past but in the lives and experiences of the individuals and families from which we descend.

THEORY

Though it may not be possible to ever be completely objective, Bowen's view, that the subjectivity inherent in psychoanalytic theory was a major obstacle in moving toward a science of human behavior, was central to his effort. In the scientific sense, theory generally includes some facts as well as suppositions about what might be factual. Though it includes subjectivity, theory is constructed to exist apart from human subjectivity. It serves as a framework for the exploration of natural phenomena with a goal of incorporating new facts as they are discovered. If a theory of the family were to become scientific and open to knowledge developing in the sciences, Bowen believed it would have to be based on systems thinking and in the human as a product of evolution. Systems thinking would be required both to account for the complex reciprocal processes occurring in the family and to incorporate knowledge from all levels in the sciences pertinent to behavior, from genetics to physiology to psychology. Indeed, systems thinking would appear to be required of science at all levels of study (Shapiro, 2011).

Basing the family in the context of evolution also contributed to an increase in objectivity. A valid theory represents the facts of an area of study along with conjectures about what might eventually become factual. A valid theory must also be consistent with the known facts discovered in the sciences. At this point in time, evolution can be considered to be a fact, even though many of the processes involved in evolution remain theoretical, that is genic versus multilevel selection. Viewing the human as an evolved form of life would be required if a theory were to be grounded in biology and what is factual about life on our planet. A common view in psychology, at the time that Bowen was formulating his theory, was that the human was unique and different than other forms of life, that our elaborate brain placed us in a separate category. Bowen saw it differently and wrote,

> One basic view that has influenced my thinking since the 1940s is that man is an evolving form of life, that he is more related to lower forms of life than he is different from them, that most psychological theories focus on the uniqueness of man rather than his relatedness to the biological world, and that the instinctual forces that govern all animal and protoplasmic behavior are more basic in human behavior than most theories recognize. (Bowen 1978, 270)

Grounding the theory in systems thinking, evolution, and biology, left it open to the facts developing in the life sciences which add to its future development and either support, modify, or reject it.

Murray Bowen considered the concept of "emotional objectivity" to be one of his significant contributions to the field. His use of the term "emotional" was quite different than its more common use of the word. It is most commonly used to be synonymous with a feeling. Merriam-Webster's Dictionary (2020), for example, defines emotion as "a conscious mental reaction (such as anger or fear) subjectively experienced as strong feeling usually directed toward a specific object and typically accompanied by physiological and behavioral changes in the body." Bowen defined the family as an emotional system to place it in the context of evolution and to place the automatic functioning of the unit and its members in the context of the automatic, instinctual behavior existing in all of life's many forms. More basic than the feeling system, which requires a nervous system and a level of brain complexity, the emotional system, in Bowen's view, is basic in all of life's almost four-billion-year history. In defining the family as an emotional system, a natural system among natural systems, Bowen made a quantum leap in the observation of human behavior and how it might be conceptualized.

Bowen's concept of the emotional system establishes human behavior in its evolutionary context. In describing his development of his theory, Bowen (1978) wrote,

> There were some basic assumptions about man and the nature of emotional illness, partially formulated before the family research, that governed the theoretical thinking and the choice of the various theoretical concepts, including the notion of an "emotional" system. Man is viewed as an evolutionary assemblage of cells who has arrived at his present state from hundreds of millions of years of evolutionary adaptation and maladaptation, and who is evolving on to other changes. In this sense, man is related directly to all living matter. In choosing theoretical concepts, an attempt was made to keep them in harmony with man as a protoplasmic being. . . . There are emotional mechanisms as automatic as a reflex and that occur as predictably as the force that causes the sunflower to keep its face toward the sun. I believe that the laws that govern man's emotional functioning are as orderly as those that govern other natural systems and that the difficulty in understanding the system is governed more by man's reasoning that denies its existence than by the complexity of the system. (p. 158)

A basic premise in Bowen theory is that the evolution and functioning of the family exist independently of how the human thinks about the family. Bowen believed that the science of human behavior would someday become a reality. The future will determine how far science can go in the effort to move toward emotional objectivity. The advances occurring in the neurosciences in recent decades, along with other scientific disciplines, have been rapidly moving in that direction. Bowen theory and the concept of the emotional system, which will be further discussed in the next two chapters, would appear to provide a conceptual framework for the integration of knowledge. In the next chapter, I would like to discuss some of the knowledge developing in the neurosciences which I think will lend some support to the concept of differentiation of self and the adaptive capacity of individuals.

Chapter 3

The Brain and Self-Regulation

The human brain is undoubtedly one of the marvels of nature. The rapid expansion of the brain found in Homo sapiens over a relatively brief period of evolution has been remarkable. With over 30 billion neurons in our neocortex alone and more than a million billion interactive connections between these cells, it represents a quantum leap in complexity from that of our nearest living primate relative, the chimpanzee. The greatest expansion of not only size but the complexity of neurons occurred in the prefrontal cortex (PFC) (Elston, 2003; Fuster, 2002).

This amazing evolutionary development has clearly been advantageous for our species, evidenced by Homo sapiens' capacity to survive and reproduce in most of planet Earth's environments, a phenomenon described as ecological dominance (Flinn & Alexander, 2007). But not all of life's creatures have depended on a central nervous system (CNS) or brain to effectively adapt to their environments. As previously mentioned, for the greater part of life's history on Earth, organisms did not require a CNS to seek nutrients, avoid predators or toxins, store information, and reproduce (Allman, 1999). The initial single-celled organisms were able to maintain an internal homeostasis in relation to the environment. Under threat they could pull together with others to form colonies which further enhanced their adaptive capacity. Neuroscientist Antonio Damasio at the University of Southern California nicely describes this adaptive capacity in bacteria in writing:

> Bacteria are very intelligent creatures: that is the only way of saying it, even if their intelligence is not being guided by a mind with feelings and intentions and a conscious point of view. They can sense the conditions of their environment and react in ways advantageous to the continuation of their lives. Those reactions include elaborate social behaviors. They can communicate among

themselves—no words, it is true, but the molecules with which they signal speaks volumes. The computations they perform permit them to assess their situation and, accordingly afford to live independently or gather together if need be. There is no nervous system inside these single-celled organisms and no mind in the sense that we have. Yet they have varieties of perception, memory, communication, and social governance. The functional operations that support all this "intelligence without a brain or mind" rely on chemical and electrical networks of the sort nervous systems eventually came to possess, advance, and explore later in evolution. (Damasio, 2018 p. 54)

The complexity of life significantly increased about 2 billion years ago with the emergence of cells with a nucleus and other organelles. This unit is believed to have been the result of a symbiotic merger of what had previously been free-living unnucleated cells (Margulis, 1981). The merger represented a quantum leap in the evolution of life forms allowing this new aggregate to adapt to increasing levels of what had once been a toxic substance—oxygen. In another billion years, multicellular organisms consisting of nucleated cells emerged and the pace of evolution accelerated. The growth in the complexity of multicellular species, from sponges to invertebrates with nervous systems to brained vertebrates, required increasingly sophisticated mechanisms to regulate the stability and integration of their complexity. As neuroscientist Joseph LeDoux (2019) writes,

As animals became more complex, consisting of multiple cell types organized into systems, new challenges were faced in terms of maintaining the integrity of the organism as a self-sustaining unit in which the parts sacrifice their individuality to maintain the physiological viability of the whole. The nervous system was the solution. (p. 124)

Later, as more complex organisms evolved, the nervous system became more elaborate with the emergence of brains. More complex brains co-evolved with more complex organisms enabling their required regulation and assisting in their adaptation. Neuroscientist Joaquin Fuster (2013) captures just one neural system involved in the brain's amazing role in automatically regulating our physiology:

Deep in the mammalian brain, between the two cerebral hemispheres there is a structure named the hypothalamus—because it lies under the thalamus, the major relay station for sensory pathways on their way to the cortex. The hypothalamus harbors a collection of tightly packed nuclei devoted to the regulation of a large variety of basic physiological functions, such as temperature, heart rate, response to stress, and endocrine functions ranging from body metabolism to growth, ovulation, lactation, blood sugar, and so on. . . . Without fail, every one of the regulatory functions of the hypothalamus, which for good reason can be called the *organ of homeostasis*, makes use of chemical or neural *feedback* to correct and stabilize the internal milieu. (pp. 88–89)

And the hypothalamus goes beyond its regulatory function with our internal milieu to play a role in such behaviors as feeding, sex, bonding, flight, and aggression.

In addition to its homeostatic regulatory functions, the evolution of nervous systems and the brain entailed an increase in memory and learning. This led to increasing flexibility in the capacity to respond to a changing environment. Behavior became less automatic as organisms could learn from experience and modify their behavior in responding to environmental challenges and opportunities.

Homo sapiens, having the most complex brain of any animal, is the fortunate recipient of this evolutionary development. Our large brains allow us to process complex information about the environment, to store relevant information, to anticipate future scenarios, and to respond on the basis of these processes. Our complex brains permit the use of sophisticated language and so to communicate and expand our knowledge. Humans are inherently social and our elaborate cognitive, linguistic, and emotional processes allow us to engage in cooperative operations involving thousands of individuals such as landings on the moon and Mars. Further, we also have the ability to transmit knowledge and experience over generations, adding to the knowledge base and the potential to respond more effectively to life's challenges. Along with our sophisticated neural hardware, however, we also embody our ancestral physiology with its more automatic and reflexive patterns of responding to and with our fellow beings, and the environment. The range from life-enhancing to life-destructing behavior is all too apparent in our species.

The brain, of course, is not a stand-alone system, but part of very complex and interactive regulatory systems. Nor does the brain serve as a strictly top-down executive, directing the functioning of the other regulatory systems. Multidirectional signaling occurs at all levels among these systems as they reciprocally contribute to one another's functioning and the overall response of the organism. Further, the human brain is designed by nature to be sensitive and highly responsive to the social environment. As Gerald Edelman (2006) writes, the brain is not only embodied in the physiology of the body but embedded in its environment. The expanding field of social neuroscience provides many examples of the complex interplay taking place among our physiological substrates, our brains, and the social environment. The neuropeptide oxytocin among other biological elements, for example, influences how we view the social world (Norman et al. 2012).

In this chapter, I will discuss the brain and the peripheral physiological systems involved in an individual's adaptive response to challenges or threats. The effectiveness of these systems is central to the regulation of self and adaptive capacity. I will also discuss these adaptive systems in relation to the systems theory of the family developed by Murray Bowen. Later I will discuss how the family is seen in shaping individual differences in adaptive capacity.

REGULATORY SYSTEMS

The human brain is central to self-regulation and the adaptive capacity of individuals, but its effectiveness is based in the cooperative interactions with the body's other regulatory systems as well. For the greater part of the twentieth century, the three major regulatory systems (the central nervous, endocrine, and immune systems) were viewed as acting independently from each other, with each serving their specific regulatory functions. That was before research led to the discoveries that these systems were in communication with one another. The immune system cells were found to have receptors for neuropeptides and hormones produced in the nervous and endocrine systems. And the nervous and endocrine systems were found to have receptors for cytokines which are produced by the immune system. In responding to stress or injury, the three systems signal one another and respond to the others' signals in order to cooperatively mount a response to a potential threat (Taub, 2008). The brain influences the functioning of the endocrine and immune systems but is also influenced by them. All three regulatory systems comprise a larger coordinated system vital to the maintenance of a stable homeostasis. This process will be discussed in more details in chapter 6, but I mention it here to illustrate how highly integrated the brain is with the entire body. It is easy to see the brain as being in charge, rather than functioning as part of an integrated whole. Antonio Damasio (2010) places the brain in its evolutionary and functional context in writing:

> *neurons exist for the benefit of all the other cells in the body.* Neurons are not essential for the basic life process, as all those living creatures that have no neurons at all easily demonstrate. But in complicated creatures with many cells, neurons *assist* the multicellular body proper with the management of life. (p. 38)

The same could be said for the endocrine and immune systems, as each contributes to the overall adaptive capacity of individuals. Each is responsive to disturbances or changes which impact the homeostatic balance of the body. In responding to internal or environmental change, the regulatory systems respond in a coordinated manner to either maintain stability or mobilize the organism to effectively react. The failure to effectively respond can result in physical, psychiatric, and behavioral disorders. The brain, for example, can regulate the immune system via the HPA system through the release of the stress hormone cortisol. Cortisol serves an anti-inflammatory function by downregulating proinflammatory cytokines. The brain can also upregulate proinflammatory cytokines through the sympathetic nervous system through the release of epinephrine and noreprinephine (Shields, Moons & Slavich, 2017b). The immune system, in turn, regulates brain functioning through the proinflammatory cytokines, which are peptide signals released by immune cells. Neurons have receptors for cytokines and so the immune system can directly modulate the activity of neural systems such as the PFC (Shields, Moons, & Slavich, 2017b).

While the regulatory systems are largely automatic and occur outside of awareness, the more recently evolved higher cortical systems in the human allow for some capacity to influence these automatic processes (Shields, Moons & Slavich, 2017a). The higher cortical processes add some flexibility of response to internal and external stimuli. For example, the sight of a dog may trigger the fear response in a person based on an earlier experience. While this response may be automatic, a thoughtful assessment and a conscious effort to engage dogs over time can allow a person to override this response. Individuals vary in their capacity to modify their automatic responsiveness. Bowen theory posits that the family plays a central role over the course of development in shaping the degree to which individuals can utilize higher cortical systems in regulating self and in responding to environmental challenges.

BOWEN THEORY AND THE BRAIN

The interconnectedness of the brain is observed not only in relation to the internal workings of the body but in relation to its social environment as well. The brain evolved and develops in a family relationship system (Allman, 1999). Our altricial beginning and lengthy development require the protective environment of prolonged parental care. From infancy on, individuals learn to adapt to their family and in that context learn to adapt to the wider social world. The brain is the central organ system connecting our physical interior with the external environment and the family is the central social environment influencing its development.

Murray Bowen's observation that the family functioned as a unit and shaped variation among its members in their adaptive capacity led to his positing that three systems were at play: the emotional system, the feeling system, and the intellectual system (Bowen, 1978). Though biological processes were assumed to underlie all three systems, their existence was inferred from the observation of behavior. It was the functioning of the emotional, feeling, and intellectual systems and not their physiological structures that Bowen described. All three systems were posited to be involved in the regulation of behavior. Knowledge developing in the sciences, especially those involving neuroendocrine processes, has shed light on the biology involved in behavior (Sapolsky, 2019) and has contributed to the further development of Bowen theory. A discussion of the emotional, feeling, and intellectual systems and some of the neuroendocrine processes involved will hopefully contribute to an understanding of the interplay between brain and family functioning.

THE EMOTIONAL SYSTEM

The use of the term "emotional" varies among investigators in the neurosciences and can lead to some confusion. In its popular use, "emotions" and "feelings" are generally used interchangeably and this is also the case for many in the neurosciences. Other neuroscientists differentiate between the two. A brief survey of several prominent neuroscientists will not adequately depict the depth and complexity of their work, but it does illustrate the range of differences in how these terms are used.

Psychologist Lisa Feldman Barrett (2017), who developed a constructionist theory of emotion, largely equates feelings and emotions. Emotions/feelings such as fear, sadness, and anger are not viewed by Barrett as having a universal basis in human nature, but rather as constructed within the brain and shaped by previous experience and the culture. Barrett also posits that particular neural systems for emotions/feelings do not exist, but that feelings are constructed by the highly integrated processing of the entire brain. Her use of the term "emotion" does not include the more basic processes Bowen includes in the term, but her research provides interesting findings related to the "feeling system" defined by Bowen (Galloway, 2020).

For the purpose of research, neuroscientist Joseph LeDoux (2015; 2019) adheres to a view that the study of emotions should only include feelings and that they cannot be inferred to exist in other animals as feelings require consciousness. He writes,

> For me, the subjective experience—the feeling—*is* the emotion. These are not hardwired states programmed into subcortical circuits by natural selection, but rather cognitive evaluations of situations that affect personal well-being. They thus require complex cognitive processes and self-awareness. (LeDoux, 2019 p. 200)

In the study of animals, LeDoux uses terms like "arousal" and "motivation" in place of "emotion" to describe certain internal states.

A contrasting view is found in the work of Jaak Panksepp (1998), a pioneer in the study of emotion. Based on his research, primarily with nonhuman animals, he viewed most animal species as experiencing emotions. Panksepp viewed emotions as having a neural basis and involve instinctual states derived from our evolutionary past. He writes,

> A central, and no doubt controversial, tenet of affective neuroscience is that emotional processes, including subjectively experienced feelings, do, in fact, play a key role in the causal chain of events that control the actions of both humans and animals. . . . In other words, emotional states arise from material events (at the neural level) that mediate and modulate the deep instinctual nature of many human and animal action tendencies, especially those that, through simple learning mechanisms such as classical conditioning, come so readily to be directed at future challenges. (Panksepp, 1998 p. 14)

Panksepp thus viewed emotions as serving adaptive functions emerging during our mammalian evolutionary history. Subjectively experienced feelings, according to Panksepp, exist in higher order animals and not just the human. He posited that mammals have a "sentient self" and thus can experience feelings of rage, fear, play, and lust. He viewed that the later evolved and more complex higher cortical systems found in the human allow for a fuller and more extended awareness of feelings and even some capacity to regulate behavioral responses. This potential for an increase in awareness provides the human with the capacity for greater flexibility in adapting to the environment according to Panksepp.

Neuroscientist Antonio Damasio (2018) shares Panksepp's view of the mammalian heritage of our emotions in writing:

> Our natural behavioral tendencies have guided us toward a conscious elaboration of basic and nonconscious principles of cooperation and struggle that have been present in the behavior of numerous forms of life. Those principles have also guided, over long spans of time and in numerous species, the evolutionary assembly of affect and its key components: all the emotive responses generated by sensing varied internal and external stimuli that engage appetitive drives— thirst, hunger, lust, attachment, care, fellowship— and recognizing situations that require emotional responses such as joy, fear, anger, and compassion. Those principles, which as noted earlier are easily recognizable in mammals, are ubiquitous in the history of life. (p. 22)

Similar to Bowen, Caltech neuroscientist Ralph Adolphs (Adolphs & Anderson, 2018) believes it is important to make a distinction between emotions and feelings, seeing feelings as representing the conscious experience of emotions. He believes that a science of emotions can occur and would need to include behavior, psychology, and neuroscience. In contrast to LeDoux, he believes such a science would need to include the study of species from worms to people.

Antonio Damasio (2010; 2018) and Joaquin Fuster (2002; 2013) also differentiate between emotions and feelings. Both see emotions as being based in the brain and body. Fuster (2013) refers to both the structures and functions of emotion. He writes,

> Like the substrate of cognition, the substrate of emotion is amply distributed, this one mainly in the subcortical regions. It has two major components: the sensing or feeling of emotion, and emotion itself, which, as the etymology of the word indicates, has a "motor" element.

In describing the feeling and behavioral components and their distribution throughout the body, he continues,

> The sensing and feeling component resides in the limbic brain, the orbital prefrontal cortex, and the receptors and nerve endings of the autonomic nervous system, scattered throughout the viscera and their ducts. The "e-motional" cerebral substrate resides in the same structures, mainly in their output or "motion" side—that is, their output side—which modulates emotional expression, blood flow to the skin and other organs, and the drives of instinctual (phyletic) origin—sex, flight, feeding, and aggression. (p. 102)

In discussing the human, Damasio makes a similar distinction between emotions and feelings in writing:

> Emotions are complex, largely automated programs of *actions* concocted by evolution. The actions are complemented by a *cognitive* program that includes certain ideas and modes of cognition, but the world of emotions is largely one of actions carried out in our bodies, from facial expressions and postures to changes in viscera and internal milieu. Feelings of emotion, on the other hand, are composite *perceptions* of what happens in our body and mind when we are emoting. (Damasio, 2010 p. 109)

Given the differences in the use of the terms, it is easy to understand how they might be misinterpreted. Developing his systems theory prior to the findings of much of recent neuroscience, Murray Bowen fell on the side of distinguishing between emotions and feelings, defining emotion as basic to all forms of life. Based on his observation of the behavior of individuals and families, Bowen's description of the emotional, feeling, and intellectual systems is remarkably consistent with a range of current views in the neurosciences. The definition of these terms, however, varies among neuroscientists as well as what is believed should be included or excluded in science. Bowen defined the three systems as functions underlying human behavior, with the assumption they have a basis in biology. He did not, however, ascribe these functions to specific neural structures. Basic human functioning, from severe dysfunctions, such as that found in schizophrenia, to optimal levels, was conceptualized by Bowen as based in what he defined as the emotional system. He writes,

> The theoretical assumption (of Bowen theory) considers emotional illness to be a disorder of the *emotional system*, an intimate part of man's phylogenetic past which he shares with all lower forms of life, and which is governed by the same laws that govern all living things. The literature refers to emotions as much more than states of contentment, agitation, fear, weeping, and laughing, although it also refers to these states in the lower forms of life – contentment after feeding, sleep, and mating, and states of agitation in fight, flight, and the search for food. For the purposes of this theory, the emotional system is considered to include all of the above functions, plus all the automatic functions that govern the autonomic nervous system, and to be synonymous with instinct that governs the life process in all living things. (Bowen, 1978 p. 356)

In basing the family and behavior in evolution, Bowen conceptualized the concept of the emotional system to refer to the basic processes underlying all life. This would include the functioning of individual microbes aggregating into a colony as well as the functioning of the microbial colony itself. It would include the differentiation of cells during development in multicellular organisms as they migrate to take up their position to function as specialized cells, as well as the functioning of the larger animal of which they are a part. Stated more generally, the emotional system as conceived by Bowen involves all those automatic processes at play in the functioning and regulation of living systems from genes to cells to individual organisms to social groups. Complex brains, from this perspective, represent an expression of an evolutionary process selected for due to their contribution to the enhancement of adaptive capacity, to their success in survival. As Damasio (2010) writes,

> Life and the conditions that are integral to it—the irrepressible mandate to survive and the complicated business of managing survival in an organism, with one cell or with trillions—were the root cause of the emergence and evolution of brains, the most elaborate management devices assembled by evolution, as well as the root cause of everything that followed from the development of ever

more elaborate brains, inside ever more elaborate bodies, living in ever more complex environments. (p. 60)

The concept of the emotional system by Bowen extends beyond the automatic and instinctual functioning of individuals to include the functioning of the social or relationship systems. And while much of brain functioning is seen as automatic and based in the emotional system, the emotional system is not limited to neural processes. The feeling and intellectual systems, however, do involve the higher cortical systems.

THE FEELING SYSTEM

Murray Bowen in defining the emotional system as including all of the automatic processes underlying the functioning of life included all that might be considered instinctual plus all of the automatic responsiveness of an organism acquired through experience. Thus it includes all that one inherits genetically and epigenetically from the previous generations, as well as learned behavior. And again, learning is found among all species from microbial forms to mammals.

The evolution of more complex brains led to an increased capacity to respond less automatically. The ability to store more experience in memory permitted organisms to modify their behavior in response to environmental changes. This capacity does not require consciousness as Eric Kandel (2006) so beautifully described based on his research with sea snails. However, the more highly developed brains found in the human, as well as some other animals, permitted an increased level of awareness. Our elaborate brains give us the potential to be aware of some of our automatic emotional responses. We can, for example, be aware of having a fear response to a situation such as public speaking or of being attracted to someone we find appealing. Our brains also evolved to be aware of and respond to the feelings of others. It is this conscious awareness of an aspect of the emotional system that Bowen defined as the feeling system. He described it as the link between the emotional and intellectual systems allowing for the awareness of emotional processes. He writes, "The emotional and *feeling systems* are interconnected, each influencing the other. The *feeling system* is a bridge between the emotional and intellectual systems through which subjective states from the upper levels of the emotional system are registered in the cerebral cortex" (Bowen, 1978 p. 423).

Decades later Damasio, who I doubt had any knowledge of Bowen theory, described feelings in a similar manner.

Feelings are mental experiences, and by definition are conscious; we would not have direct knowledge of them if they were not. But feelings differ from other mental experiences on several counts. First, their *content* always refers to the body of the organism in which they emerge. Feelings portray the organism's interior—the state of internal organs and of internal operations—and, as we have indicated, the conditions under which images of the interior get to be made and set them apart from the images that portray the exterior world. (Damasio, 2018 p. 102)

Early in his research Bowen observed that people vary in the degree to which they could distinguish between their thoughts and feelings. An example of this was found among the families in the NIMH research study when a concern about a health issue arose. Bowen observed that the mother, father, and adult schizophrenic child were unable to distinguish between a feeling that an illness existed and the fact of whether it did or not (Bowen, 2013). The feeling of being sick was taken as evidence of an illness. This contrasted with the relationships between the parents and the other siblings, in which they could be more objective. In a report about this observation Bowen wrote,

In summary, the functioning of a series of families about health matters is characterized by an intense emotional process in which the mother, father and child are deeply involved with one another. Thinking about health issues is heavily in the service of feelings, with marked impairment of objectivity and of effective action. The impairment is apparent whether the difficulty is a physical or an emotional one; the distinction between the two is regularly blurred, and one mistaken for the other. (Bowen, 2013 p. 128)

The observation that the thinking and feelings "blurred" together in the parents and their adult child with schizophrenia appears to have been one of the many significant discoveries by Bowen during the Family Study Project. He observed the variation among other siblings who were able to be less "subjective" or feeling oriented with regards to a concern about an illness. The feelings and facts were less blurred for them. The study of this observation was expanded by Bowen with less impaired outpatient families and others, as he sought to find a dimension along which individuals varied in their adaptive capacity. Eventually this observation became a central element in his concept of differentiation of self. Individuals functioning at higher levels of maturity were found to have the capacity to distinguish between their thoughts and feelings and, as a result, more choice in whether to base their decisions and behavior in a more thoughtful or less feeling-based manner. Individuals, on the other hand, who functioned at lower levels of adaptiveness, could not make this distinction and their lives were directed more in a feeling-based way. Bowen developed the concept of the intellectual system to describe the higher cognitive processes involved in varying degrees by individuals in regulating their behavior and in directing their life course.

THE INTELLECTUAL SYSTEM

The brain is central to self-regulation, allowing us to maintain a stable internal homeostasis in the face of environmental changes. Large-brained animals generally have longer life spans, have greater capacity to process incoming information, and have greater capacity to store experience with an enlarged memory. The emergence and evolution of ever more complex brain structures and functions led to increasing levels of plasticity in the capacity of organisms to self-regulate and respond to environmental stimuli. The more automatic processes involved in self-regulation long preceded cognition and are amazingly elaborate.

Conserved by natural selection, the automatic neural processes underlie the most sophisticated manifestations of human existence, shaping our lives and behavior more extensively than we are generally aware of. Evolution's gift of an increased capacity for cognition, enabled by the expanded neocortex and its elaborate PFC, is built on a foundation of the earlier evolved brain and nervous system and is intricately embedded in the brain and body.

One of the clearest examples of the degree to which higher cortical systems such as the PFC remain embedded in older and more automatic regulatory systems is that of the stress response system. The autonomic nervous system (ANS) and the hypothalamic–pituitary–adrenal system (HPA) are activated in response to perceived internal or external threats and designed to upregulate and downregulate the physiological systems needed to effectively respond such as the fight, flight, or freeze responses to environmental threats as well as other neuroimmune-endocrine system responses to internal threats. Given the primacy of survival, these evolutionarily older systems take precedence over the higher cortical systems in the face of threat. While the higher cortical systems function in reciprocal relationship with the more automatic emotional processes, during heightened stress the subcortical systems predominate (Panksepp, 1998).

The upward subcortical signals, for example, are active in downregulating the PFC under stress (Arnsten, Wang, & Paspalas 2012; McEwen 2007; Raio et al. 2013) and in decreasing its influence in regulating the emotional system. Neural connections are always bidirectional (Silvers, Buhle, & Ochsner, 2013) and information arriving at the PFC has already been processed in the associative, sensory and motor cortices, and in limbic systems such as the thalamus and amygdala. Information is not simply relayed by these systems;

their processing is colored by previous experience and by the hormonal and ANSs to which they are connected.

Our elaborate brain exhibits its evolutionary history over the course of development. The prenatal assembly of the brain unfolds in a manner similar to its phylogenetic history, with the more recently evolved brain structures developing later. This process continues throughout the course of development. In an interactive process, the genetic blueprint and experience together shape both the structures and functions of the brain. A process that includes myelination, pruning, dendritic growth, and a resculpting of synapses is experience dependent and active throughout adolescence (Fox, Levitt, & Nelson, 2010).

The integration of our higher cortical systems with the brainstem and limbic system in reciprocal feedback processes provides us with the capacity to have some conscious awareness of the more automatic responsiveness of these systems. And though our thoughts, feelings, and behavior may be more determined by the instinctual responsiveness of our evolutionary heritage than we like to admit, we have also inherited the potential to observe and to some degree regulate or modify our responses to the environment. As Damasio (2010) writes,

> The difference between life regulation before consciousness and after consciousness simply has to do with automation versus deliberation. Before consciousness, life regulation was entirely automated; after consciousness begins, life regulation retains its automation but gradually comes under the influence of self-oriented deliberations. (p. 176)

Individuals vary in the extent to which their behavior comes under the "influence of self-oriented deliberations," but this capacity represents a significant evolutionary advancement in self-regulation. Deliberate thinking entails reasoning and logic. It expands the capacity for choice and adds another level to our flexibility in adapting to the environment. In what appears to be unique to the human, the expansion of the PFC allows not only for the potential to enhance an individual's adaptiveness to the current environment, it enables the consideration of the future. Neuroscientist Joaquin Fuster (2013) captures this extraordinary development:

> The human brain retains from evolution, as a matter of fact, all of its reflex apparatus to adapt to the external and internal milieus and to correct for changes in both. But in addition, it becomes capable of anticipating those changes and of preparing the organism for them. Whereas in past evolution the mammalian brain became adaptive by natural selection, the human brain, in addition, has become *pre-adaptive*. (p. 24)

Being integrated with the various subcortical and bodily systems, the PFC provides an individual with the potential to reflect on one's self-in-the-environment, to have memories of past experience, and to project into the future. All of which can allow us to have some choice in how we might respond to our life situation. It is this capacity to have some choice in how we respond to life's challenging situations and in directing one's life course that determines the adaptive capacity of individuals.

Murray Bowen's observations and his conceptualization of the range of levels of maturity evident in human functioning led to his development of the concept of differentiation of self. He viewed the adaptive capacity of individuals to vary along a continuum, varying in degree but not in kind. This was a significant departure from mainstream psychiatry. It eliminated the categorization of much of human functioning into discrete diagnostic categories. Instead, he viewed individuals as varying from those at the lowest levels of adaptiveness to those who appeared to function at the highest levels.

In defining the intellectual system Bowen (1978) writes:

> The intellectual system is a function of the cerebral cortex which appeared last in man's evolutionary development. . . . The cerebral cortex involves the ability to think, reason, and reflect, and enables man to govern his life, in certain areas, according to logic, intellect, and reason. . . . The feeling system is postulated as a link between the emotional and intellectual centers through which certain emotional states are represented in conscious awareness. (Bowen, 1978 p. 356)

The maturation or differentiation of the intellectual system over the course of development is evidenced in the degree to which it can be utilized in both self-regulation and self-determined behavior during stressful periods and in emotionally important relationships. Though it is seen as a function of the cerebral cortex, like most brain functions the intellectual system entails a host of interacting cortical and subcortical systems. As mentioned earlier, it describes a function more specific than cognition.

The concept of differentiation of self describes the variation among individuals in their adaptive capacity. It posits that the interplay, observable in behavior, between the emotional and intellectual systems varies based on the differentiation of the intellectual system. It reflects both a developmental process and a level of functioning. The differentiation of a self and related differentiation of the intellectual system is seen as central in determining the basic stability of an individual's functioning over a life course. Bowen described this interplay in writing:

> This (differentiation of self) has to do with the way the human handles the intermix between emotional and intellectual functioning. At the highest level are

those with most "differentiation" between emotional and intellectual functioning. They are more free to live their emotional lives to the fullest, or they have
the capacity to make decisions based on intellect and reasoning when confronted
with reality issues. People at the lower levels have emotion and intellect so
'fused' that intellectual functioning is submerged in emotionality that their lives
are dictated by emotionality. (Bowen, 1978 424)

Those individuals demonstrating a greater level of "fusion" between the
emotional and intellectual systems can be observed to have less choice or
flexibility in how they respond to significant challenges. Their behavior is
based more on automatic, internal responsiveness to environmental stimuli,
than on a more realistic appraisal of the current environment. Given their
heightened responsiveness to the relationship environment, their life course
is less self-directed and more influenced by others. They find it more difficult
to tolerate the tension states which often accompany life transitions. Their
behavior will more likely be directed toward obtaining feelings of comfort
and avoiding the challenges which may result in short-term stress but can
result in long-term gains. Individuals with a lower level of maturation or differentiation in their intellectual system have a lower capacity to self-regulate
in emotionally important relationships. Their own emotional functioning
tends to be more regulated by others and in periods of stress they are more
vulnerable to withdraw or engage in conflict. As a result, relationships will
be less likely to serve as potential resources.

Individuals with a more developed or differentiated intellectual system
have both a greater capacity to be aware of their automatic emotional responsiveness and more choice in how they respond. They have more latitude in
assessing whether their automatic response would be adaptive or whether
other options would be more effective or beneficial to themselves and others.
Bowen observed that individuals who functioned at higher levels of differentiation were able to use their intellectual system to arrive, over time, at basic
principles and beliefs which they could rely on to guide their behavior during
more stressful periods when the feeling system was more predominant. They
had a greater capacity to remain engaged with important others during periods when emotional reactivity in the relationship system was running higher.

A frequent misunderstanding of the concept of differentiation of self is that
"emotions" are viewed as negative in Bowen theory and "intellect" is positive. Such a view misses the point that the emotional system, as defined in
Bowen theory, is seen as vital to life and as underlying our adaptiveness and
self-regulation. It is predominant in our lives. Differentiation of the higher
cortical systems, however, simply provides us with the capacity for some
choice. The automatic works fine for the most part, but it can also at times
lead us to respond in a manner that is maladaptive.

As mentioned earlier, the subcortical systems are more predominant especially during stressful times or situations. A principal variable influencing the "intermix" of emotional and intellectual functioning is the level of anxiety. More on the influence of this aspect of adaptive functioning will be presented in chapter 6 in which the impact of stress on the family will be discussed. Bowen made the distinction between the functional level of differentiation of self of individuals and their basic level. Shaped over the course of development, one's basic level is seen to be established at a stable level by young adulthood. One's functional level, however, can fluctuate to some degree from their basic level due to fortunate or unfortunate fluctuations in their environment. During periods of prolonged stress, for example, an individual's level of stress reactivity or chronic anxiety may increase and thus influence their level of functioning. Similarly, prolonged periods of positive regard from others in a relationship system may boost an individual's level of functioning.

At the present time, it is not clear to what extent a person's basic level can shift during adulthood. It does appear that a conscious determined effort by an individual to increase their basic level to some degree is possible (Bowen, 1978; Kerr, 2019). A structured approach in this effort is described in chapter 10. An assessment of whether an upward or downward shift has occurred, however, is difficult based on the number of variables needed to be considered; that is, length of time the functioning is sustained during both fortunate and stressful periods, the functioning of important others in one's relationship system, and so on. Most changes in functioning are seen as occurring in one's functional level and not the basic level of differentiation.

Much remains to be learned regarding the neurobiology of differentiation of self. It can be assumed that genetic, epigenetic, physiological, psychological, and relationship factors are involved (Bowen, 1988). Since the time in which Bowen developed his theory of the family system, a wide range of knowledge emerging in biology and the neurosciences have shed light on the reciprocal influence which occurs among these factors (Arnsten et al., 2012; Carter, 2005: Champagne & Curley, 2015; Cole, 2013; Ellis et al., 2011; Fox et al., 2010; Fuster, 2003; Lupien et al., 2009; Meaney, 2010; Nusslock & Miller, 2016; Porges, 2011; Taub, 2008).

The process of differentiation of self is seen as being both enhanced and constrained by the family emotional system. Differentiation develops in the day-to-day and year-to-year interactional processes occurring in the family. Much remains to be learned about this process involving biological, psychological, and relationship variables as they interact with one another, but Bowen theory posits that as a higher-level unit of biological organization, the family is involved in regulating this process. The family system, then, is central to the development of differentiation attained by offspring and that variation in the maturity of individuals is shaped within each family and over the generations. In a 1976 interview, Bowen described some of the complexity involved in the family's shaping of an individual's basic level of self:

> On another level it would be accurate to say your differentiation level is deter-mined by the differentiation level in your parents at the time you were born, your sex and how that fitted into the family plan, your sibling position, the normality or lack of it in your genetic composition, the emotional climate in each of your parents and in their marriage before and after your birth, the qual-ity of the relationship each of your parents had with their parental families, the number of reality problems in your parents' lives in the period before your birth and the years after your birth, your parents' ability to cope with the emotional and reality problems of their time, and other details that apply to the broad configuration.

He goes on to say:

> In addition, the level of differentiation in each of your parents was determined by the very same order of factors in the situation into which they were born and grew up, and the levels of differentiation in each grandparent was determined by the same factors in their families of origin, on back through the generations. As I see it now, the biological, genetic, and emotional programing that goes into reproduction and birth is a remarkably stable process, but it is influenced to some degree by the fortunes, misfortunes, and fortuitous circumstances when things go wrong. All things being equal, you emerge with about the same basic level of differentiation your parents had. (Bowen, 1978 p. 409)

In this quote, Bowen clearly places the differentiation of a self in a multigenerational context. It is a context consisting of the interactions and functioning of members of the generations preceding one's parents and their environmental challenges during the births and development of their offspring. Many might see this as highly deterministic, but the variable of differentiation includes varying degrees of choice in each generation. The context of one's life is greatly expanded in this view. It certainly belies the often mischaracterization of the concept of differentiation of self as an indi-vidualistic concept.

It is in family interactional processes, occurring over the course of devel-opment that the intellectual system develops the capacity to function along-side the feeling system or the degree to which it is overridden by it. It is in this context that individuals develop their responsiveness to others and the degree to which they regulate self or are co-regulated in the relationship system.

And the context of an individual's development is placed in a context of the interdependent development of others.

The evolution of brains in the animal kingdom allowed for the enhanced regulation of more complex bodies and for an increased capacity to adapt to changing environments. The neural systems most vital to the regulation of our physiology and survival develop first beginning in prenatal development and early postnatal infancy. For the human, the social environment has been central and the more recently evolved structures and functions of the human brain with all of their complexity appear to have evolved due to the selective advantage they offer individuals in navigating our complex social environments (Dunbar, 2002; Flinn, 2005). The PFC develops the most and the latest over the course of development (Fuster, 2002) and appears designed to assist individuals in learning about and adapting to the current environment. In order to adapt most effectively in the social arena, the individual must not only accurately assess that environment, but learn to regulate his or her more automatic emotional responsiveness in the midst of it. The intellectual system as defined in Bowen theory involves more than the PFC, but it is central to its functioning and in the development of the adaptive capacity of individuals. The principal context for the development of the self-regulating system of the brain is the family. The brain is embedded not only in the body but in the family emotional system and the differentiation of the intellectual system occurs, according to Bowen theory, within the context of the family adaptive system.

A woman I had met with several years previously regarding her family called recently to request a consultation. She described a phone call she had with an adult son the previous week. He lived in another city and she said she called him weekly. She mentioned that it took some work on her part as he was not highly communicative. "On our calls, I am dancing as fast as I can to keep the conversation going," she said. She was proud of this son and took some pride in maintaining their relationship. She requested a consultation following a conversation in which he said he did not think she had been a particularly good mother to him. "It broke my heart," she said. He was due to come home the next weekend for a family gathering and she had asked him if they could get together for coffee to discuss his view further. In our session, we discussed her relationship with this son, the current state of the larger family, and what she hoped to accomplish in their meeting. We scheduled another appointment following her coffee with the son.

In our next meeting, she described a positive visit with this son. During their discussion he mentioned that one of the problems he had with her was that in their weekly phone calls he felt like he could never get a word in. "I could see that in my anxious effort to connect with him, I hardly left any room for him." She said she now saw one of the ways she could be problematic in their relationship. She realized that if she could better manage her anxiety about their relationship and not feel fully responsible for it, it would likely go better. She knew she had to learn to inhibit her own amount of talking and learn to take the time to listen to him. She became clearer that they each played a part in how they related and she now had a better sense of how she might manage her part more effectively.

I thought this was a fine example of the emotional, feeling, and intellectual systems at play in this relationship. The emotional system was reflected in the underlying connectedness between mother and son, with each responding automatically to one another. Her emotional involvement led to an anxious effort to engage, while his led to an anxious retreat. Her feeling system involved feeling rejected and having "a broken heart." And the mother's intellectual system wanted to understand the process. She could see a pattern she had not seen before and could decide to modify her behavior in that context with her son.

The emotional, feeling, and intellectual functions are not, of course, entirely separate. They are functions of a highly integrated brain. At their most effective, they can operate as a team as they process the signaling transpiring across the various neural systems involved. But the emotional system with its automatic responsiveness has a greater capacity to override the intellectual system. With sufficient stress this occurs for all, though the extent to which this occurs will vary based on the differentiation of the intellectual system. In the larger population, there is variation in the capacity of individuals to utilize their intellectual systems in emotionally important relationships and in response to stressful events. According to Bowen theory, the family is the context in which this capacity develops. Though he is not specifically referring to the family, biologist Gerald Edelman (2006) nicely described the variation in brain functioning and its basis in both evolution and development when he wrote,

Inasmuch as a large portion of brain development is stochastic and epigenetic— that is, is strongly influenced by the fact that neurons that fire together wire together—no two brains, even those of twins, are identical. Thus, in analyzing the structure and function of the human brain, detailed history must be taken into account, first during evolution and then during individual brain development. (p. 55-56)

The evolution of the cerebral cortex in the mammalian line occurred in the context of increasingly prolonged and engaged parental care and in the human involved the coevolution of the reproductive unit of the family. The increasing complexity of the brain also permitted an increase in the complexity of the social environment beyond the family (Dunbar, 2016). The prolonged development of the brain and its ability to effectively regulate emotions and behavior are central to the adaptive capacity of individuals in the increasingly complex social organization occurring over hominin evolution. During the course of adolescence, the myelination or white matter of the brain is increasing and the pruning of gray matter in the PFC continues into young adulthood. Over the long course of development, the "firing and wiring" of neural circuits principally occur in the highly integrated and patterned relationship environment of the family.

Bowen theory posits that the family emotional system to a significant degree is central in shaping the maturation or differentiation of the higher cortical systems involved in an individual's capacity to self-regulate and develop a self-directed course in life. The family has been observed to be more than a collection of individual personalities. It is seen as a highly regulated system which generates variation in the adaptive capacity of its children. I think most would acknowledge how central the family is in the development and well-being of people. What has been more difficult for most to see is the degree to which the family is involved in the ongoing regulation of behavior. Getting beyond the view of individuals as entities separate from their family relationship systems appears to be more difficult for most to observe. The level of interdependence at play in the functioning of families and their members and the degree to which it shapes their behavior has not yet been widely accepted. Bowen theory posits that relationship patterns developed in the family form the basis for how individuals function in their future family and social relationship systems.

Chapter 4

The Family as an Adaptive System

The experience early in my career of meeting with families in their homes as an alternative to the hospitalization of one of their family members who had become psychotic or suicidal provided a foundation for the observation that families operate as highly interdependent systems. It became clear that the thoughts, feelings, and behaviors of individuals were being significantly governed by the interactional processes occurring in the family. Over a span of three years, I was afforded the opportunity to meet with families who were going through periods of heightened stress. At such vulnerable times, families are generally quite open as they seek relief from their anguish. And meeting with them in their own homes provided an additional level of openness in discussing their experiences.

Initially the families were understandably focused on their symptomatic member as each member described what they saw as a build-up in the intensity of the distress of that member and the family. Their view, similar to the one prominent in the mental health field, was that the symptoms reflected only the dysfunctioning of the individual family member. After hearing their concerns, family members were asked about the period leading up to the development of their member's breakdown. Asking "how, what, when, and where" questions led to three remarkable observations.

First, in backing up from their immediate fears and describing events occurring both within the family and in the broader context of their lives, it became clear that the family had been experiencing a particularly stressful period for the family. The death of a grandparent, a job loss, or other changes affecting the family were usually described. It appeared evident that the decline in a family member's functioning was occurring in the context of this prolonged period of heightened stress. The family, and not just the individual, was adapting to the stressful events they described.

A second observation was that as family members began to thoughtfully describe the troubling events in their lives over the previous months or year, the emotional intensity in the family usually began to decrease. And more remarkably, as the family tension began to subside, so did the intensity of the symptoms of the identified troubled family member. Although this did not always occur in the first sessions, there was in general a sense of relief that perhaps the family could manage to keep the symptomatic member at home. Once the tension or anxiety in the family began to decline, their functioning began to improve. The linkage between family functioning and the emergence and severity of symptoms seemed obvious to me.

The third observation occurred due to the involvement of extended family members in the therapy sessions along with gathering information about changes in the larger family. It became clear that the nuclear families were not entirely separate from the extended family or from the events which impacted them. Often, an important change in the extended family, such as a death or the diagnosis of a life-threatening illness, was not seen as related to the functioning of the symptomatic person. It is difficult during a crisis, for example, for most families to see the death of a grandparent occurring eight months prior to the development of a symptom in the immediate family as related. Once it became clear how emotionally interconnected members of the nuclear family were to the larger family, it was easier to see that a disturbance in the balance of relationships in the extended family could have a profound effect throughout the family.

The observation of the interlinked functioning of family members during especially stressful times was an eye-opening experience. Certainly, it became evident that the symptomatic family member generally fared better when they could remain in the family rather than being extruded to an institution. It was also convincing that the larger extended family was an important part of a nuclear family's functioning, that the more isolated families had a more difficult time recovering. A figure/ground shift occurred in observing that the family could be a resource to the symptomatic member and that the engagement of the extended family could have beneficial effects for the nuclear family unit. The family sessions did not resolve the underlying difficulties for the symptomatic member of the family. They did, however, reduce the family tension and as a result the intensity of the symptoms. After the family therapy sessions in the home, the families were referred to a community mental health center.

I followed the experience with family crisis intervention team by taking a position in an outpatient drug abuse treatment program. Initially the program principally involved heroin and amphetamine addicts. At the time family therapy was rarely utilized in the treatment of this population. In taking the position, I reasoned that if the family was indeed central in the development of symptoms, it should apply to the individuals who became addicted as well. I began including family members in the therapy and found that the addicts, most of whom were in their 20s, appeared to be highly dependent on their families, and especially involved with their mothers. I did a survey of 323 drug addicts in the program (Noone & Reddig, 1976). Seventy-two percent (average age 24.4) either lived with their families of origin or had in the previous year. A great majority were in daily contact with their mothers. This was contrary to the then accepted view that most addicts had rejected their families.

The years of treating addicts and their families reinforced the view that families operated as interdependent systems. Both the families and the addicted members generally were unaware of this interdependence. Parents saw their young adult sons or daughters as rejecting their families and the addicts typically saw themselves as independent of their family's influence. A common view held by the families at that time was that their sons' or daughters' addictions were principally due to the negative influence of their peers. Observations of the family relationship interactions, however, belied their stated opinions. The dependence on drugs appeared to be related to the reciprocal dependence between the parents and their adult son or daughter. The addicts' siblings usually functioned better and were more emotionally independent of the parents. The underlying challenge faced by these families seemed to be related to the difficulty they had in both adapting to recent stressors as well as the difficulty the parents and symptomatic son or daughter had in separating and moving into adulthood. The emotional involvement was generally most intense between the addict and the mother. Socioeconomic factors were also relevant, but they were not enough to account for the functioning of these symptomatic families. Families from upper socioeconomic levels were also observed to exhibit similar patterns and symptoms. It was not only the young adult drug addict but the family that appeared to lack the adaptive capacity to address their current life challenges.

Despite the rich opportunity in observing families and immersing myself in the growing family systems literature, I grew dissatisfied with my own growth in developing the capacity to "think systems." A variety of conceptual frameworks had emerged in the family therapy field (Guerin, 1976). Each provided a way of moving from an individual paradigm to a family systems paradigm and permitted me to see a new level of complexity governing behavior. Each of the various frameworks I had studied consisted of underlying assumptions which attempted to account for both what kind of system the family is and what its interactional processes entailed. The observation of families convinced me that "systems thinking" was required to understand the complexity involved. Operationally, however, I found myself reverting to "individual thinking" during family therapy sessions. I could know intellectually that a family functioned as an integrated system but found myself either taking sides with a member in seeing him or her as being victimized or focusing on one member as the "problem." After a session, I could regain a systems perspective, but I was frustrated at not being able to maintain it during an emotionally charged meeting.

While attracted to a number of systems approaches, it became apparent to me that I lacked a coherent conceptual framework. I realized that the mixture of conceptual frameworks could not be integrated and that their use actually became an obstacle to clearer thinking and observations on my part. After six years of working with families, I decided to become more grounded in one approach in the effort to speed up my learning. At the time I chose the theoretical approach which had been developed by Murray Bowen at NIMH and Georgetown University. The decision was based on two primary considerations. Bowen's family systems theory (later known as Bowen theory) entailed a multigenerational perspective of the family, which at that point in my work seemed vital. My previous work with inner-city families highlighted the fact that nuclear families were a part of a larger family process. Bowen theory was also the only approach which included a method for making gains in one's own family, another aspect of working with families I viewed as vital.

Regarding the first consideration, the experience of observing three-generational families highlighted the influence previous generations had on the functioning of families in the present. The teaching of family therapist and psychiatrist Carl Whitaker (Neill & Kniskern, 1982), who had emphasized the importance of the extended family and had earlier been a consultant to the hospital program I was involved in, also played a part in the decision to study Bowen theory.

The second consideration in choosing to become grounded in Bowen theory was related to the importance I attached to become knowledgeable about my own family and the part I played in it. The inability to observe my own family as a system along with little detailed knowledge about my extended family and history was apparent to me. I had been making such an effort but had made little progress. I could observe clinical families functioning as systems with repeating relationship patterns, but I was unable to have much clarity about this in my own family of origin. This observational blindness was a motivating factor. I knew that my own functioning was influenced by my family, but I didn't quite know how. I assumed that my own immersion in my family played a big role in my inability to see.

At the time I entered the postgraduate training program at Georgetown, however, I did not have a clear idea of what a formal theory entailed and was unaware of the central role the natural sciences could play in my understanding of the theory and families. The recognition of the value of a formal theory in science and the value of viewing human behavior in the context of evolution were exciting developments which I saw as greatly expanding my potential for learning. Just as the observation of families and the introduction to family systems thinking allowed me to see what I had not seen before, the natural systems theory of the family developed by Murray Bowen opened a new vista. It was a vista that led to an interest in the natural sciences and evolution and an expanded view of the human family. I slowly came to grasp that theory was central to the scientific effort and that if a theory were to remain open it would need to be open to and consistent with the facts and knowledge being acquired in the sciences.

ORIGINS OF A NEW THEORY OF HUMAN BEHAVIOR

Early on, Bowen's primary objective was to see to what extent a science of human behavior could be developed. There had been some discussion in psychiatry about whether psychoanalysis could become scientific. As he became trained in psychoanalytic theory and psychotherapy, this question was being raised in the field (Rakow, in press). While he was at the Menninger Foundation, Bowen began the then unorthodox practice of meeting with the families of those hospitalized with schizophrenia. Contrary to psychoanalytic thinking of the time, he thought it would be useful to learn more about the families of the patients. Since it was unconventional at that time, he began meeting with the families in the evenings and on Sundays. He also wrote letters to the families informing them about the status of their hospitalized family member (Rakow, in press). His observations led him to conclude that rather than undermining treatment, contact with the family could be a resource to the treatment.

By the time Bowen began his Family Study Project at NIMH in 1954, he had already begun to develop the concepts of differentiation of self and the emotional system (Kerr, 2019; Rakow, in press). He already had a view of the importance of family and a view that the problems evidenced by those with severe mental illness existed in all people, though in varying degrees.

Once the fathers and siblings began to live on the research unit, a new set of observations was made by Bowen and the research staff. From its beginning, the research project was based on a process of developing hypotheses and then modifying them when they did not match the observations. As Bowen wrote in a summary of the five-year project:

> The research study was started in 1954. The initial working hypothesis had been developed several years before during the course of individual clinical work with schizophrenic patients and also with their mothers. The hypothesis

considered schizophrenia to be a psychopathological entity in the patient which had been influenced to a principal degree by the mother. It considered that the basic character problem in the patient, on which schizophrenic symptoms are later superimposed, was an unresolved, symbiotic attachment to the mother. The initial focus of the study was on the mother-patient relationship. (Bowen, 1978 p. 47)

The hypothesis was tested by seeing the schizophrenic patient and the mother separately in psychotherapy and then predicting how they would interact with each other. Initially the fathers did not live on the unit. They would, however, visit on the weekends and the impact of their visits could be observed. Based on these observations, the fathers and siblings of the patient were invited to join their families in living on the unit. This led to observations which had not been expected and led to a change in the original research hypothesis.

It was now hypothesized that the mother–offspring relationship represented only an element or fragment of the larger family. Once the nuclear families living on the ward could be observed on a day-in, day-out basis, a new order of phenomena not previously seen was observed. As Bowen wrote,

A number of facets of the human phenomenon come into view in observing family members together that are obscured with any composite of individual interviews. Any person who exposes himself to daily observations of families as they "relate to" and "interact with" each other is confronted with a whole new world of clinical data that do not fit individual conceptual models. (Bowen, 1978 p. 152)

The research highlighted the level of interdependency and reactivity found among the family members and led to the observation of repeated interactional patterns. Once these patterns could be observed in the families living on the research unit, the same patterns could more easily be observed in the outpatient families. Among the early observations by Bowen was the "stuck togetherness" at play among family members. The fluidity of anxiety or tension as it moved from one member to another was evident. Early on in the project he wrote,

The most striking (observation) was the fluid, shifting character of the mother–patient attachment. It was more than a state of two people *responding* and *reacting* to each other in a specific way but more a state of two people *living and acting and being for each other.* There was a striking lack of definiteness in the boundary of the problem as well as lack of ego boundaries in the symbiotic pairs. The relationship was more than two people with a problem involving chiefly each other; it appeared to be more a dependent fragment of a larger family group. There was this quality referred to as "transfer anxiety" in which the anxiety or sickness or psychosis could shift from one to the other, or to other family figures or, to a lesser degree, to staff members. (Bowen, 1978 p. 10)

The fluid nature of anxiety in the research families led to the observation of what Bowen described as "the emotional oneness within the family" (Bowen, 2013, p. 108). After the first year of the study, the research hypothesis was changed to a "family as a unit" hypothesis. Observations of the process of schizophrenia shifted from seeing it as an individual phenomenon to seeing it as a phenomenon involving the whole family. Similarly, the research observations led from a focus on the mother–child dyad to the family. This represented a dramatic departure from conventional thinking.

This shift, from viewing the behavior of family members as based on the fixed characteristics of individuals to one in which their behavior could be seen as an interactive process was described by Bowen:

Before this experience (after fathers and siblings were admitted to the research unit) we had thought in terms of "the father *is* one kind of person, the mother *is* another kind of person, and the patient *becomes* another kind of person." The research operation had first gone toward defining what we believed to be the fixed characteristics of each family member. After we had seen changes in one family member followed by immediate complementing changes in other family members, and after we had seen changes in characteristics formerly considered to be fixed, we began to work toward the concept of the functioning of one person in relation to another. (Bowen, 1978 p. 29)

Following the observations that the family functioned as a unit and engaged in repeatable interactional patterns, the concept of the nuclear family process was developed. Seeing the family functioning as a system led to the question of what kind of system is it. As mentioned previously, Bowen believed that a theory of behavior, if it were to move toward science, had to be placed in the context of evolution, as a part of all life. In grounding the human as a product of evolution, Bowen conceptualized the family to be an emotional system. The term "emotion" is often confused with "feeling," but Bowen defined it as a process basic to all life.

The emotional system, as defined by Bowen, refers to a process universal to all life, including forms of life predating the emergence of nervous systems and brains. Basing his observations and the proposition that the human and his or her behavior are representative of an evolutionary process contributed to Bowen's ability to see that the behavior of individuals and families is largely automatic and operates outside of awareness. Defining the family as an emotional system grounded human behavior in this basic ancestral process.

It is interesting that others have similarly described the regulation of complex behavior by social groups prior to the evolution of vertebrates. In using the term "emotion" in a manner similar to Bowen, Damasio (2018) writes,

> Social governance has humble beginnings, and neither the minds of *Homo sapiens* nor of other mammalian species were present at its natural birth. Very simple unicellular organisms relied on chemical molecules to *sense and respond*, in other words to detect certain conditions in their environments, including the presence of others, and to guide the actions that were needed to organize and maintain their lives in a social environment. (p. 19)

And in another description of complex behavior occurring in "mindless" bacteria, Ben-Jacob et al. (2011) write,

> As a member of a superorganismic colony, each bacterial unit (cell) possesses the ability to sense and communicate with others. Together they constitute a coordinated collective that performs integrated tasks in communication with others. Collective sensing and cooperativity are intrinsic to microbial communication. Multicellular superorganisms (communities) generate in their constitutive elements (individual bacteria) new traits and behaviors not explicitly stored in the genes of the individuals. (pp. 56–57)

The very earliest of life forms then had the capacity to merge into more complex relationship systems, which then function in a manner not reducible to the sum of their individual members. Although human behavior is far more complex, the example of bacterial colonies does capture the phenomena defined by Bowen in his use of the term "emotional system." Automatic adaptive behavior exists in all forms of life, with the human not being an exception. Similar to bacterial colonies and other more advanced relationship systems comprised of individual entities, the human family can be observed to collectively respond to its environment.

In referring to the basic homeostatic processes of the family, Michael Kerr (2019) refers to the original work of Claude Bernard and Walter Cannon:

> Bernard's and Cannon's basic idea is that unicellular and multicellular organisms have physiological processes that maintain a constant balance or equilibrium regardless of changes in their external environment. Any tendency toward change in that constancy automatically meets with factors that resist the change. The adaptive capacities of unicellular and multicellular organisms attempt to preserve this state of equilibrium. The concept of homeostasis applies to the

human body, and by viewing the family as a unit—an organism in its own right—it is possible to consider a family as a homeostatic system as well. For example, disturbances in the family relationship system trigger automatic emotional reactions to restore the balance. (p. 305)

In addition to family members adapting to one another and the environment, each family unit itself can then be seen as an adaptive system. This process is observed to be largely automatic and operating outside of the awareness of its members. Central to all forms of life is the maintenance of an internal stability or homeostasis. The survival and reproductive success of organisms at all levels of complexity require the maintenance of a stable internal milieu. Such stability requires regulatory mechanisms that are activated when the balance of this milieu is altered. As life forms evolved to become more complex, so too did the regulatory mechanisms required to maintain this complexity in relation to the environment. The mammalian brain is an example of a complex system that evolved in part to regulate the larger multicellular system of which it is a part. Bowen theory posits that the human family represents such a form of evolved complexity with its own regulatory mechanisms (Papero et al., 2018).

The observed interdependence of family members involves a significant degree of sensitivity to one another, such that a change in one member predictably results in a compensatory change in another. The co-regulation observed in families is more than a psychological process. While emotional reactivity in relationships can be observed behaviorally, its influence can also be observed at the physiological level as well (Buchanan et al., 2012; Butler & Randall, 2013; Harrison, 2020). When a change results in a disturbance in the interactional balance or homeostasis of the family system, automatic mechanisms are activated to restore the previous balance of functioning.

The greater the level of emotional dependency at play in a family, the more sensitized members are to each other, and the more their functioning is regulated by one another. Greater sensitivity among members results in their being more emotionally reactive to each other, especially under stress. Sensitivity as described here refers to the automatic responsiveness individuals have to each other and not to a conscious awareness of each other's emotional functioning. Another way of saying this is that, at higher levels of differentiation, family members have a greater degree of emotional autonomy and a greater capacity to self-regulate in emotionally important relationships. This allows them to put less pressure on the others in order to manage themselves and to be less vulnerable to being regulated by the other family members.

In recent decades there has been substantial evidence supporting the observation that relationships are vital ingredients in the regulation of the physiological, emotional, and behavioral functioning of individuals

(Butler & Randall, 2013; Carter, 2005; Cacioppo & Patrick, 2008; Uvnas Moberg, 2003). It is important to note, however, that for the most part such studies have largely remained based on what might be called an individual paradigm. Dyadic relationships and even group relationships might be described, but the focus remains on the reciprocal influence individuals have on one another in a dyad. The view of the family as a higher order self-regulating system regulating the functioning of its members is absent.

The "oneness" or undifferentiation is less pronounced in more adaptive families, and less energy is utilized by members in reacting to one another while under stress. The members of more adaptive families exhibit a greater capacity to realistically assess the threats posed by particular stressors, resulting in less of what might be called "stress contagion" (Buchanan et al. 2012). Being less reactive to the stress reactivity of other family members can allow one to more effectively respond to them and to the stress at hand. In being less reactive to others, they have a greater capacity to be present and to act as a resource (Kerr & Bowen, 1988; Papero, 2015). Emotional reactivity is not absent among families at higher levels of differentiation, but in having more access to higher cortical systems (intellectual system) during stressful periods, individuals have more latitude in whether their behavior is determined by their automatic emotionality or whether they have some choice to respond differently.

At lower levels of differentiation, individuals are more responsive to and regulated by the emotional signaling occurring among family members. Less differentiated families exert more emotional pressure on one another in responding to stress and to one another. The pressure can take the form of expectations of one another or blaming. For example, a mother who has had a stressful day at work may respond by emotionally "shutting down." Her husband, sensitized to his wife's emotional functioning, perceives her as being distant to him and as a result becomes tense and irritated. Going into the next room, he sees his son playing video games and reacts with irritation, telling him to turn it off and do his homework. Son reacts negatively and the tension and voice levels increase between the two. Mother hears the squabble and reacts by admonishing her husband as being too harsh with their son. Husband and wife then get into conflict about their son and father leaves the room angry at both.

This scenario, of course, can take place in any family, depending on the level of stress one or more members may be experiencing. Families exhibiting greater levels of "oneness" or fusion, however, are more sensitized to one another and have less capacity to regulate their emotional reactivity. With regards to the emotional reactivity presented in this example, it will take less stress to trigger reactivity in a family with less differentiation, the reactivity will be more intense, and it may persist for a longer time. In a family with a lesser degree of "oneness," the same process of reactivity might occur, but the members will have more ability to manage their reactivity to one another resulting in a less intense and shorter period of reactivity.

Relationships are a basic element in how people regulate their functioning. A difference, however, is the extent to which one is dependent on others to regulate their functioning. The process of maturation can be viewed as an increasing capacity to self-regulate. From infancy to young adulthood this process is related to brain development as individuals learn to master new behaviors and take on more responsibility. The process is also related to the relationship process in the family as individuals mature and attain greater or lesser levels of self. Bowen theory lays out many of the variables accounting for the variation in the maturational process and in the ability to self-regulate.

In the above example, mother's "shut down" will have less influence on her husband when their levels of differentiation are higher. Being less emotionally fused, father will be more likely to observe that she is stressed and as a result take her stress response of shutting down less personally. Since he is less emotionally dependent on his spouse, her stress will not as likely be experienced as threatening to him. Rather than react to her "shut down," he may be better able to assess whether to approach and inquire about her stress or whether she just needs some space. His ability to regulate his emotional response results in the initial stress being less contagious and he in turn will have a better chance of managing his reaction to his son more effectively. The more emotional oneness in a family, the more emotional contagion will be at play in tense situations.

It is a premise in Bowen theory that all families exhibit a level of family "oneness," but the level of basic differentiation or undifferentiation will vary among its members based on a family's position in the multigenerational family emotional process and an individual's position in the family (Bowen, 1978). The level of oneness or togetherness increases for all families when its homeostatic balance is disturbed, resulting in an increase in emotional reactivity among its members. Bowen posited that the equilibrium of a family or other relationship systems appears to be maintained by two counterbalancing forces which are influenced by stress or increases in tension. He writes,

> A relationship system is kept in equilibrium by two powerful emotional forces that balance each other. In periods of calm, the forces operate as a friendly team, largely out of sight. One is the force for togetherness powered by the universal need for emotional closeness, love, and approval. The other is the force for individuality, powered by the drive to be a productive, autonomous individual, as determined by self rather than by the dictates of the group. (Bowen, 1978 p. 311)

As a living system, the family is in a constant process of adapting. The disturbance of a family's homeostasis predictably results in the activation of regulatory mechanisms which result from the members adapting to one another as well as the unit's adapting to the environment in which it lives. From the perspective of Bowen theory, the family emotional system entails all levels of complexity from genes to physiology to psychological processes to the relationship system. In adapting to the environment, these systems can be involved in reciprocally interacting with each other; all can be seen as contributing to the ongoing balance of a family's functioning.

FAMILY ADAPTIVE PATTERNS

A family's homeostasis entails the interactional patterns that have been established over time. While each member is actively participating in those patterns, the functioning of the family unit represents more than the sum of the individuals' behaviors. In the effort to both be connected and maintain autonomy, individuals attempt to influence the behavior of each other. Each member, regardless of age, can be seen as seeking to maintain a degree of internal comfort or equilibrium. When periods of calmness prevail, it is easier for members to be reasonably comfortable. It is a quiet process as members relate to one another and maintain a balance of connectedness and autonomy. Members exert minimal pressure on one another during such periods and experience little pressure from the others as a stable balance is maintained. In a sense, each has more "space to be." Each can move toward another without encroaching on the "self" of the other. As a dynamic living system, however, change is inevitable, and the family and its members will need to adapt. Adaptations are required in response to the life cycle challenges of births, illnesses, job and locations changes, deaths, and so on. They are also required when the environment presents a family with new challenges such as an economic recession or other societal events. The basic interdependence at play in the family is highlighted during periods of change when members are responding to both the change and the responses of one another to the change.

The birth of a child is a good example of the adaptations required by all the members of a family. It is usually a welcomed event, but the functioning of every family member is affected. Hormonal changes are occurring principally for mother but also for father and grandparents (Flinn, Ward, and Noone 2005). Neuroscientist Stephen Porges, in describing what he calls the "symbiotic regulation" between mother and infant dyad, writes,

> The caregiver becomes part of a complex feedback system supporting the biological and behavioral needs of the infant. Within this model of symbiotic

regulation, the caregiver is not solely giving to the infant. The behaviors of the infant also trigger specific physiological processes (e.g., neural and endocrine feedback circuits) that help establish strong bonds, provide emotional comfort for the caretaker, stimulate neural pathways, and support the health of the caregiver. (Porges, 2011, p. 281)

Mother and infant's emotional involvement goes beyond the dyad and requires a rebalancing of the emotional system. A sibling may be displaced and has to adapt to no longer being "number one." Even though he might be delighted with this new family member, father will experience a shift in the marital emotional involvement as mother responds to the infant. The energy demands on both parents are substantial. In effect, the family will never be the same. The former homeostasis is disturbed as each member adapts not only to the infant but to each other's adapting to the infant and to one another. The development of a new equilibrium requires change.

While all families necessarily adapt to such significant changes, the range of how well families adapt varies significantly. According to Bowen theory, variation in the adaptive capacity of families is related to two principal factors: (1) the level of differentiation of self existing in the family unit and (2) the level of chronic anxiety the unit and its members are experiencing. The two factors are related to one another, though the level of chronic anxiety is more likely to fluctuate in relation to significant stressors, while the basic level of differentiation of self is a stable characteristic of individuals. More regarding chronic anxiety will be discussed in chapter 6.

Differences both within and between families can be observed in the degree of interdependence they exhibit, but at a basic level this variation does not vary widely within individual families. The chapter on the family multigenerational process will describe how a wide range in the adaptive capacity of families develops over the generations, but in each generation the level of adaptive capacity of siblings is principally determined by the level of differentiation of the parents and the family's interactional patterns. Siblings may vary in this characteristic, but each child will predictably attain a level varying only in degree from that of the parents.

A premise of Bowen theory is that in the process of courtship and marriage, people tend to select partners at similar levels of emotional maturity. And this basic level of maturity establishes a baseline for their children as they develop. Growth and the movement toward maturity is an intrinsic characteristic of individuals, but it principally occurs in the context of the family.

The degree of emotional dependence individuals retain over the course of their own development will shape the establishment of family oneness in the next generation. It is "as if there is a certain amount of 'immaturity' to be absorbed by the family system" (Bowen, 1978 p. 167).

The concept of the nuclear family emotional process in Bowen theory describes four emotional patterns or adaptive mechanisms utilized by families in maintaining a balance over time. The extent to which the mechanisms are used is based on the basic level of emotional autonomy/dependence (differentiation) of family members and the stress or challenges they face. In a sense the family interactions observed when these mechanisms are activated can be seen as efforts in both self- and other-regulation by the family members and the family system itself.

In describing the four mechanisms, or emotional patterns as Kerr (2019) describes them, I will be using nuclear family examples. The mechanisms, however, can be observed in all relationship systems. Distancing, conflict, reciprocal over- and under-functioning, and triangling are adaptive processes evident in all emotional systems (Bowen, 1978; Kerr & Bowen, 1988; Papero et al., 2018).

The relationship parents have with their families of origin is another variable influencing the frequency and degree to which the adaptive mechanisms or patterns are activated. During periods of stress, the family will be more stable when the parents have maintained emotional contact with their original families. When a family is more isolated from the extended family during stressful periods, the mechanisms will be called into play to a greater degree. Families more isolated or emotionally distant from their families of origin become more emotionally dependent on each other. As a result, the sensitivity and emotional reactivity in the unit will increase. As I will discuss in chapter 8, the levels of maturity or differentiation of self play a significant part in the capacity of individuals to remain in contact with the extended family. Individuals with lower levels of maturity are more vulnerable to emotionally cutoff from the extended family and as a result are less able to benefit from their potential resourcefulness and less capable of being a resource to the extended family.

The mating process, occurring during courtship and in making the long-term commitment of marriage, is shaped by the levels of maturity each partner has attained in their families. Early in the relationship, as they settle into an "emotional oneness," the connectedness is usually experienced as rewarding. In addition to the psychological sense of well-being resulting from the closeness they experience, the biological substrates involved in attachment are at their most active stage (Uvnas Moberg, 2003). It is predictable that after some time couples will create a certain level of emotional distance in their relationship. This appears to assist the pair in managing the sensitivity and reactivity they have toward one another due to the fusion which inevitably has occurred. There is a cost to the new unit they have formed, for the fusion or merger has also resulted to some degree in a loss of autonomy. The distance which develops is an adaptive process which can add to the stability of the relationship. It is both a result of the sensitivity or reactivity the couple has developed toward one another but also a way to decrease the reactivity. The degree of emotional distance they establish will be determined by the level of fusion or dependence created in the new unit.

One of the costs incurred in the marital fusion is a decrease in the level of openness a couple can maintain in their relationship. The level of fusion is determined by the level of differentiation they bring to the relationship. At lower levels of differentiation, they will become more emotionally dependent on one another and more sensitive to the reactions of the other.

During courtship, most couples exhibit a good deal of openness with each other. They share thoughts and feelings more readily. At this point in their relationship, even with their strong attraction, they are more separate individuals. A stable fusion in the relationship usually takes place once they have committed to a long-term relationship. With the resulting increase in emotional dependence, the well-being of each also becomes more dependent on the other. There is an increase in emotional contagion as an increase in anxiety in one will likely trigger an increase in anxiety in the other. The greater their levels of differentiation, the more they are able to maintain some degree of emotional autonomy. Paradoxically, the greater degree of emotional autonomy in the marriage allows for more openness in a relationship. Emotional autonomy permits partners to be more present to one another. Being less emotionally dependent on the other for their well-being, they are less threatened by their differences or the distress the other may be experiencing.

Individual differences, for example, will be experienced as more threatening when the level of fusion or undifferentiation is greater. Differences, which may have seemed to be attractive during the courtship, may now be seen as irritating or unacceptable. Curiosity about what the other thought may now shift to pressuring the other to think differently about a subject. Or one may suppress a differing viewpoint so as not to trigger a negative reaction in the other.

Distancing

Over the course of the relationship, distancing will be one of the adaptive mechanisms couples utilize in the effort to decrease the tension they experience when the balance of the relationship is disturbed. In response to stress, a couple will experience an increase in tension as they respond to one another. The increase in tension results from a disturbance in the individuality/togetherness balance established in the relationship. The disturbance of the balance or homeostasis in all emotional systems, be they work, family, or other relationship systems, results in an instinctual movement toward more togetherness, much like a herding response. This can have a calming effect in the short term, but over time the increased togetherness creates tension, which in turn leads to an increase in emotional reactivity. This process can be observed following tragic events in a community. The initial response of pulling together is a natural one and usually adaptive as people assist one another. After a period, however, the "crowding" results in some discomfort and people act to restore the distance which had previously existed.

In a marriage, the increased togetherness in response to stress is similar. The more emotionally dependent a couple is, the more togetherness is sought. The result is an increase in reactivity as the dependence is experienced as a kind of pressure on self from the other as well as the other's response to the pressure self puts on the partner. The increase in fusion leads to an increase in the sensitivity each has to the other. The resulting discomfort or tension they experience occurs automatically. Distancing can help to restore the individuality/togetherness balance the couple had previously maintained, resulting in a decrease in tension for the couple (figure 4.1). When more exaggerated, however, one or both partners may interpret the distance as a lack of caring. Each may see the other as more distant and see the distancing as intentional. One or both may at times seek to overcome the distance in their relationship, but it will usually be short-lived due to the fusion they share. An increase in stress for either increases the sensitivity they have to tension in the other and so each distances in order to be more comfortable.

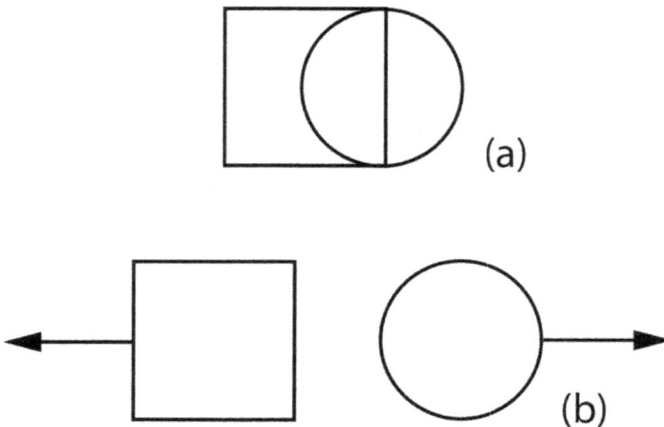

Figure 4.1 Emotional Distancing. (a) Depicts Fusion between Partners in a Marital Relationship. (b) Depicts Emotional Distancing as a Mechanism to Decrease Tension Resulting from Fusion. *Source:* Created by the author.

Less distancing is required for couples with greater levels of differentiation or emotional autonomy. They have a greater capacity to self-regulate and as a result need less distance to maintain their own emotional equilibrium. Though there may be some emotional reactivity due to an increase in tension, they will have a greater capacity to recognize their own tension and/or tension in the other and be less likely to blame self or the other. They may be aware that some distance will be useful until they are calmer. The distance will be more short-lived. As a result, each can be more present and available as a resource to the other while going through a stressful period.

Distancing, as with all four of the mechanisms described in Bowen theory, is adaptive to a point. When the mechanisms become more exaggerated or prolonged, they can be maladaptive and result in the development of symptoms or the dissolution of the marriage. Too much emotional distance for individuals can lead to an increase in emotional isolation, a breeding ground for symptoms (Cacioppo & Patrick, 2008).

For the most part, emotional distancing in a marriage generally operates outside of awareness. As Kerr (2019) writes,

> The example of one person reactively distancing and the other person developing a symptom is one of the most important ideas in Bowen theory: one person's anxiety can express itself in another person's symptoms. The anxiety transfer is not mystical. Distancing gets communicated in subtle and not so subtle ways. Anxiety-driven distancing can manifest, for example, in talking less to a partner, having less eye contact, and being more distracted. A partner can, often unconsciously, respond with an emotional reaction to having less contact that triggers that person's stress response. (p. 43)

Emotional distancing is a reciprocal process which can become the principal pattern in which each person attempts to manage the sensitivity they experience to one another in their "common self." A not uncommon comment of one or both partners seeking to end a marriage after years together is that "we have grown apart." That is accurate from a subjective, feeling point of view, but paradoxically the distancing is enacted to manage the fusion in the relationship. Over time as each distances to manage their own tension, the relationship becomes less open. Emotionally important issues are not discussed due to the concern that they might stir up more tension. Based on their fusion, an increase in anxiety or tension in one results in an increase in tension in the other. As the use of the adaptive function of distancing becomes more pronounced, each partner can begin to feel less connected. The recognition of the underlying process at play by one or both partners can provide a way through the impasse experienced by so many. When one partner can recognize their own part and not blame the other, he or she can begin to self-regulate their tension and avoid distancing. Since distancing, like the other adaptive mechanisms is a reciprocal process, one person can learn to modify it.

Conflict

A second emotional pattern or adaptive mechanism utilized by couples is that of conflict. Again, conflict can be found in most marriages, varying in intensity and frequency. The sensitivity couples exhibit toward one another is usually more apparent when it is expressed in conflict. As with the other mechanisms it is seen as a response to the discomfort partners experience due to the levels of their fusion and chronic anxiety. The merger of selves into a common self in a marriage entails a pressure for unity or togetherness. During less stressful periods the relationship can be harmonious. When stress increases, differences which had previously been tolerated can be experienced as a threat to self and result in an effort to pressure the other to be in agreement or to change. At a feeling level, each partner experiences the other as the source of their discomfort. From this perspective the solution is to get the other to cease their disturbing behavior.

When I asked one woman how she knows when her husband has had a stressful day, she described one of their patterns. "I can tell he's stressed because when he comes in the kitchen, he begins to scan the room for signs of disorder. He then complains that the house is a mess." When asked how she responds she said,

> It depends on whether I am stressed or not. If I've had a bad day at work, I let him have it and we're off and running. When I'm not stressed, and I can be aware that he's stressed, I don't take it personally and just let him walk through the kitchen. After a while, when he has calmed down, he returns and we can have a decent conversation.

This would be an example of mild conflict in which the woman could observe her own participation in the conflict. When stress is greater and/or differentiation is lower in a couple, neither partner is able to see self as playing a part in the conflict. The focus remains on the other and each can feel impinged upon by the other. This mechanism can result in intense conflict and is typically followed by distancing. The distancing can allow each to calm down and is followed by re-engaging. With sufficient stress or fusion, an ongoing cycle of conflict, followed by distance, and later peacemaking occurs, which can then be followed by the same cycle.

When conflict is the predominant mechanism utilized by a couple in their effort to manage the tension resulting from their fusion, it can become a characteristic of their relationship. The greater the fusion, the greater the difficulty partners have in seeing the other and self as separate. At its extreme, the feelings and behavior of each are regulated by the other. Each spouse can believe that the other is responsible for their upsetness and so blame them for creating the tension or stress. For the most part it is not the issues that are central to their conflict, but the emotional process involved as each struggles to maintain a self and be connected. Their level of emotional involvement is evident in both how reactive they are to one another and the amount of time and energy each devotes to the other.

Conflict can be adaptive in the marriage, allowing for the tension or anxiety to be externalized. When exaggerated, however, it results in each feeling controlled or victimized by the other. Each partner can feel that they contribute more to the relationship and that the other is not contributing their fair share. Though at the feeling level, this pattern is described as uncomfortable and unwanted, at the level of emotional process, it can have a stabilizing function for the relationship. Conflict can allow for a level of emotional involvement with the other and at the same time function to maintain a degree of emotional separateness as each engages in "a battle for self" (figure 4.2).

Reciprocal Over- and Under-functioning

A third adaptive mechanism observed by Bowen (1978) can appear less overt than that of marital conflict, but likewise is based on the fusion or merger into a common self. In this process, the stability of the unit is maintained with one partner assuming more responsibility or better functioning, while the other becomes less responsible or functions less well. In what Bowen described as the trading or borrowing of self, one partner takes on a role of functioning at a higher level, while the other gives up some of his or her functioning. Initially each person usually functions at about the same level. Once the merger of selves takes place, however, a shift in their functioning occurs. It is as though one cedes some of their functioning to the other, so that one will function at a better level for the two of them. It is a reciprocal process as each takes on one side of this reciprocal process. It may appear that one is more dominant or capable than the other, but in observing the relationship process over time, it may be difficult to assess which if either is the more dominant. Either one might be seen as initiating the more adequate or inadequate role, with the other accommodating by taking on a greater or lesser level of functioning.

Though either one may be more vulnerable to becoming symptomatic, in general it is the one who is most accommodating who develops a symptom. The partner who assumes the dominant or over-functioning position might, for example, become worn down and then symptomatic during a prolonged period of stress as he or she struggles to take on more responsibility. The

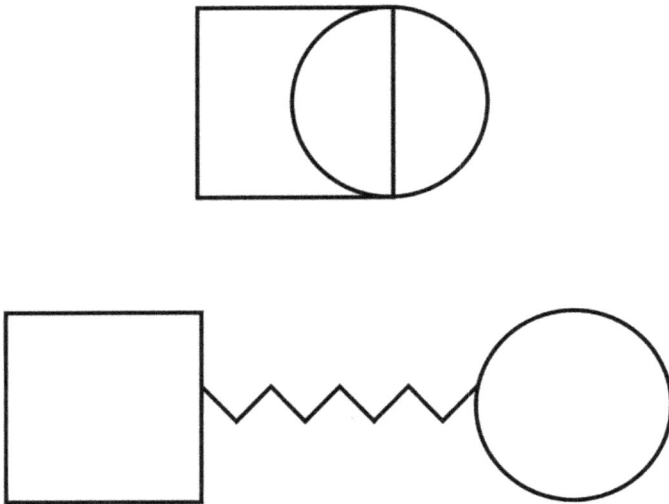

Figure 4.2   Conflict. Depicts Conflict as a Mechanism to Decrease Tension Resulting from Fusion. *Source:* Created by the author.

under-functioning partner, however, in giving up self to the other, is usually the one more vulnerable to becoming symptomatic. The over-/under-functioning mechanism can allow the partners in a common self to avoid conflict or distancing and can work well during periods when stress is at a low level. In avoiding conflict and in relying on the other to function for self, however, he or she can move into a helpless mode, feeling incapable of addressing important issues for self. With sufficient stress or loss of self, the accommodating partner can develop physical, psychiatric, or social symptoms. During periods of a family regression, this reciprocal process can take the form of one becoming more symptomatic and the other becoming the "strong one" or caretaker (figure 4.3).

This reciprocal process occurs in all families to some extent. When one partner becomes temporarily ill, for example, the other steps up to take on more responsibilities. When the level of fusion or undifferentiation is high, however, this mechanism can become predominant as each spouse becomes more "locked into" a functional position.

An example of the reciprocity involved in this pattern was described by a woman whose parents had a relationship in which her mother had been the highly responsible, over-functioning one in the marriage, while her father had a history of chronic under-employment and alcohol dependency. In her late 60s, mother developed some dementia which influenced her functioning. The daughter said, "I never would have imagined it, but my father has

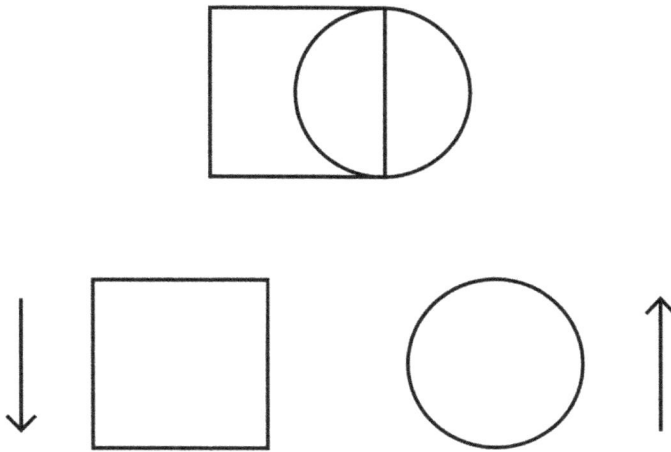

Figure 4.3 Reciprocal Over- and Under-functioning. Depicts Reciprocal Process in Functioning as a Mechanism to Decrease Tension Resulting from Fusion. *Source:* Created by the author.

become the responsible one and takes wonderful care of my mother." Another not uncommon pattern is when an over-functioning spouse dies, the under-functioning spouse pulls up their functioning.

In a fifteen-year prospective study of fifty-one marital pairs, Klever (2021) found three patterns contributing to which spouse would be more vulnerable to becoming the symptomatic one. The first entailed the reciprocal process involved in the "trading and borrowing of self" in which one spouse exhibited more purposeful self-direction and goal effectiveness. The other absorbed more of the tension and in losing self-direction and goal effectiveness became more susceptible to becoming symptomatic. The second pattern involved a "triangling" in which one spouse sided with one or more other family members in viewing the other as the problem, resulting in his or her absorbing more of the tension in the process. In the third pattern, Klever found that the marital pairs' multigenerational families could be a factor in which the spouse became symptomatic. While each is seen to be at similar levels of differentiation of self, one may have a less stable multigenerational family than the other and thus have more tension to manage in relation to his or her family.

All four of the adaptive mechanisms are more easily observed in their more exaggerated form. The over-/under-functioning mechanism was illustrated by a married couple in their late 30s. The wife was a high school principal who excelled in her profession and as a parent of their two children. The husband had developed an addiction to heroin and had been only sporadically employed during the course of their marriage. Prior to and in the early years of their marriage he had also been a teacher. During periods of heightened tension, the wife focused principally on her husband as the source of her stress and went into "overdrive" in her effort to mother and manage him. The husband became more passive and relied on drugs to manage his increased tension. For the most part the over-/under-functioning pattern in this relationship seemed to work well for this family during less stressful periods. When a significant stressful event, such as the death of the wife's father occurred, however, this pattern became more exaggerated. From a systems perspective, however, this pattern allowed the family to adapt by containing or binding the anxiety the unit was experiencing. In this case, when the wife was able to recognize her part, she began to take less responsibility for her husband's functioning and focus on defining what she was willing to do or not do. She realized that the effort she had been making in attempting to get her husband to function at a better level was unproductive and even stressful for both. Initially, the husband appeared to attempt to get her to change back into her over-functioning position, but as she maintained a position of not "functioning for him," he became less symptomatic, managing to end his addiction to heroin, and assume a more responsible level of functioning in the family.

Family Projection Process

Over the life course of siblings, their adaptive capacity can look significantly different, with one or more functioning at a fairly good level, while another functions at a significantly lower level. If Bowen theory posits that the family emotional system is central in determining the adaptive capacity of offspring, it would need to account for the disparity in functioning among siblings who have been raised in the same family. Certainly, that question was raised in the NIMH Family Study Project directed by Murray Bowen. If family emotional process was so central in the development of schizophrenia, how did other siblings appear to function so much better?

Based on the observation of families in that study, along with the study of outpatient families exhibiting less severe symptoms, the intense parental emotional involvement with one of the children was found to be the principal and consistent factor contributing to the impairment of one child and the better functioning of his or her siblings. This relationship pattern could be observed to a greater or lesser degree in all families and Bowen defined the family projection process as one of the adaptive mechanisms involved in the nuclear family emotional system (Bowen, 1978).

According to Bowen theory, each family must contend with a basic level of emotional dependence the members have on one another. As mentioned, the parents' level of maturity or differentiation creates the baseline of a family unit's emotional interdependence. It is at the heart of each family's adaptive capacity and its emotional homeostasis. The four observed adaptive mechanisms are utilized in response to a disturbance in a family's equilibrium and represent an effort to maintain the unit's oneness. Families functioning at greater levels of oneness or fusion demonstrate more frequent and exaggerated use of the mechanisms than do families exhibiting less fusion. The members of families with greater levels of differentiation are less dependent on one another for their functioning and as a result put less pressure on others to sustain their own emotional equilibrium and experience less pressure from the other members to sustain theirs.

Bowen considered the family projection process sufficiently important that he defined it as a separate concept in the theory. He believed it to be a basic emotional pattern which operates to some degree in all families. In describing the pattern he writes,

> The process through which parental undifferentiation impairs one or more children operates within the father-mother-child triangle. It revolves around the mother, who is the key figure in reproduction and who is generally the principal caretaker for the infant. It results in primary emotional impairment of the child, or it can superimpose itself on some defect or on some chronic physical illness or disability. It exists in all gradations of intensity, from those in which impairment is minimal to those in which the child is seriously impaired for life. (Bowen, 1978 p. 379)

The family projection process is one of the mechanisms which functions to stabilize the family unit. It serves to regulate the tension arising from the emotional fusion in the marital pair by triangling in a child (Bowen, 1978; Kerr, 2019). The focus on a child as a source of their tension or anxiety allows the caretakers to unite in a common concern and obviate the tension in their own relationship.

In an early observation of one of the NIMH research families, Bowen described a version of this process:

> As I currently see the mother-child equilibrium, the mother was securely in the overadequate position to another human being, this human belonged to her, and it was realistically helpless. She could now control her own immaturity by caring for the immaturity of another. With her emotional functioning more stabilized in the relationship with the child, the mother became a more stable figure for the father. He could better control his relationship to her when her functioning did not fluctuate so rapidly. He tended to establish more of a fixed position of aloof distance from the mother, similar to his relationship with his own mother. This new emotional equilibrium came to be a fixed way of functioning for the father, mother, and child. I have referred to this as the "interdependent triad." The child was the keystone. Through the relationship with

the child, the mother was able to stabilize her own anxiety and to function on a less anxious level. With the mother's anxiety more stabilized, the father was able to establish a less anxious relationship with the mother. (Bowen, 1978 p. 56; originally in Jackson, 1960)

This process is more easily identified in its more exaggerated form, described in the family discussed previously. Bowen theory posits that in the formation of a family unit, the unresolved emotional attachment or dependence each parent had with their own parents must be managed in this new family. Each parent brings a similar level of unresolved emotional attachment into the marriage and a resulting level of fusion. One or more of the adaptive mechanisms will be expressed in their relationship in the effort to reduce the tension or anxiety resulting from their fusion. The family projection process enables parents to unite in their emotional involvement with a child, diminishing conflict, distance, or symptoms in the marital pair (figure 4.4). This can take a number of forms and be expressed as positive overinvolvement with a child or excessive concern. The child is seen as playing an active part in this process. To the extent that his or her functioning stabilizes the functioning of the parents, it has adaptive benefits for the developing child. Over the course of development, however, this process serves to constrain the child's capacity to develop a more mature or separate self. The degree to which a child functions to stabilize the functioning of the parents will influence the course of his or her development. All things being considered, this child will predictably emerge from the family unit with a lower level of emotional maturity than the parents or siblings.

In a real sense, the other siblings benefit. When the family undifferentiation is more contained within a central parent–child triangle, the development of the other siblings is less constrained. The projection process can involve the whole unit in seeing one child as less capable or more problematic and become a perceived reality for all. During periods of stress and increased chronic anxiety, the focus on this child becomes more pronounced; the parental over-functioning and the child's under-functioning is more exaggerated. The family projection process, like the other adaptive mechanisms, illustrates the degree to which the functioning of its members is co-regulated within the family. The greater the level of maturity or differentiation of self that exists in a family requires less utilization of the adaptive mechanisms, but one or more of them can be observed in all families. It may take more stress in the more adaptive families for the mechanisms to be triggered, but the same patterns are a part of the basic emotional functioning at all levels of differentiation. The extent to which the mechanisms are required, however, will depend on the level of differentiation and chronic anxiety.

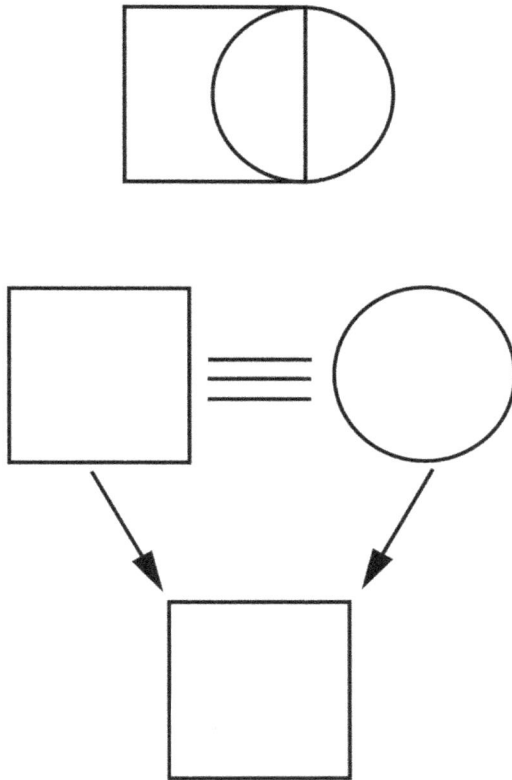

Figure 4.4 Family Projection Process. Depicts Process through Which Parental Undifferentiation Impairs One or More Children. *Source:* Created by the author.

For many it is difficult to see how these patterns can be adaptive, particularly when they may result in the development of physical, psychiatric, or social symptoms. No parent seeks to contribute to constraining the development of their child. This is not intentional behavior but an automatic process occurring at the family level of organization. What may be adaptive for the family can be maladaptive for one or more family members when the unit is overloaded.

There is a predictability about this and the other mechanisms which can be observed when the level of chronic anxiety increases in a family. The patterns repeat over and over, ebbing and flowing over the course of a family's life. The central parental triangle involved in the projection process may, for example, be barely visible during calmer times. The marital pair may relate more easily with each other. Mother may still have some concerns about the triangled child, but her focus is less intense. The functioning of the child is better both within and outside the home. It can be as though the functioning of the triangle and its members is "looser" or more relaxed. A significant event such as the death of a grandparent or an older sibling leaving home for college, however, may disturb the family balance and result in a "tightening" up of the central triangle. Father may respond to the change and resulting increase in tension with an increase in emotional distance. Along with her own anxious response to her son leaving home, mother's sensitivity to her spouse's distancing may result with an increase in her anxiety, to which both her spouse and their younger child respond. Mother may move toward her child with an increased anxious concern to which the son responds with an increase in emotional reactivity toward his mother. Mother then goes to her husband to discuss her concerns and they both engage with an increased focus on the child. This process can increase in intensity as each member responds to the others in a predictable pattern.

A systems perspective can allow the observer to see the behaviors in this family as reciprocally influential. At greater levels of intensity, the process can result in the development of a symptom in the child. This may take the form of a physical symptom such as an intestinal problem, a behavioral symptom such as school avoidance, a psychiatric problem such as panic attacks, or compulsive behavior. Absent in a systems view, the problem can be seen as existing within the child. Out of concern, this can often lead to the engagement of nonfamily members (teachers, physicians, social workers) which can further intensify the focus on the child (Brown, 2020). The involvement of professionals, with a focus on the problem as existing solely in the child, can lead to a diagnosis which often is experienced by the parents with some relief, having identified the "problem." The parents of a thirteen-year-old son who had been refusing to go to school were visibly relieved when a psychiatrist diagnosed their son as having "separation anxiety" and prescribed medication for him. The previous parental conflict, which had led to discussions of divorce, receded.

The added focus on the child can lead to solidifying the problem and not addressing the larger source of anxiety. A systems perspective, on the other hand, can allow the parents more options in addressing the increase in anxiety resulting from a change in the family equilibrium. And just as an increase in anxiety led to a process resulting in a child's symptom development, a decrease in parental anxiety due to addressing the changes in the family can lead to a decrease or end of the symptom in the child.

The four nuclear family adaptive mechanisms identified by Bowen are similar to what have been described as allostatic mechanisms (McEwen & Gianaros, 2011; Sterling & Eyers, 1988). I will further describe the concept of allostasis in chapter 6, but it refers to a process involved in maintaining an organism's homeostasis. For all life forms, homeostasis is an active process. While homeostasis refers to the stable balance of a system, allostasis refers to the processes required to maintain that stability in the face of change. Allostatic mechanisms are activated to allow an organism to adapt to change. An example would be an increase in the blood pressure needing to occur when someone is climbing stairs. Allostatic mechanisms are vital to effectively adapting to change. When allostatic mechanisms are overutilized for a prolonged period, however, it can lead to what is known as "allostatic load." This can result in a wearing down of the organism. The increase in blood pressure over years in response to prolonged stress, for example, can lead to chronic high blood pressure and the problems it entails.

Similarly, the four nuclear family adaptive mechanisms function to maintain stability in the family, but when exaggerated for prolonged periods they can lead an allostatic load on the family unit resulting in a symptom. Heightened chronic anxiety as defined in Bowen theory is an example of allostatic load occurring in a family.

Based on Bowen's view of the family as a natural system, Bowen theorist Daniel Papero (2020) has described several of the basic functions the family must serve and has developed a framework for assessing the adaptive capacity of families. Papero suggests that three of the basic functions or tasks that a family serves for its members are (1) an economic function, (2) a growth or regenerative function, and (3) a maintaining and protective function. The economic function of a family is to provide the critical resources (food, shelter, etc.) that are necessary to sustain life. The growth function of a family is to provide the context for reproduction and the development of future generations. Papero posits that the family must also provide a protective function enabling it to meet the environmental challenges which threaten a family's capacity to effectively adapt.

In light of these functions, Papero proposed a dimensional framework for assessing the adaptiveness of families. The framework consists of five continua along which families function: resourcefulness, connectedness, tension management, systems thinking, and goal structure. The model is not a measurement instrument, but a conceptual framework which can allow one to assess aspects of the overall adaptiveness of a family.

Families vary along these continua based on their basic level of differentiation and the level of chronic anxiety they are having to deal with. The position of a family on one or more of these dimensions at any given point in time will not necessarily be an indication of the family's basic adaptive capacity. During a prolonged and significant period of stress, a particular family may occupy a lower position on one or more of these dimensions than they will during more opportune periods. The use of the adaptive mechanisms by a family will also vary in the same way. It is vital to consider the context and level of stressors a family has been faced with over a period of time in order to make a more accurate assessment of their basic adaptive capacity.

Chapter 5

An Evolutionary Perspective on the Family and the Brain

In the two previous chapters, the brain and the family were presented as adaptive systems and discussed from a Bowen family systems theory perspective. In this chapter, I would like to present an evolutionary perspective on these systems. In doing so, I want to emphasize two important caveats. First is that Bowen theory is not a theory about how the human family evolved. It is a theory about how the family functions. This distinction is between what are called the ultimate and proximate levels of causation (Mayr, 1982). The ultimate level is concerned with the evolutionary history of an organism or natural system, while the proximate level is focused on how they function in the present and in their context. In developing his natural systems theory of the family, Bowen believed that if it were to contribute to a science of human behavior it had to be consistent with the facts of evolution, with the view of the human as a part of the evolutionary process with its roots in the very beginning of life. While evolution itself certainly seems to be a fact, there are a number of perspectives about how evolution operates. These are not yet facts, but hypotheses that lack sufficient evidence to be considered factual at this point in time. An example would be the question of at what level does natural selection operate. Some would see it as operating only at the genic level, others at the level of the individual, and still others as operating at multiple levels. Bowen theory is not based on any of these conceptual positions, which leads to the second distinction I would like to make.

I will be presenting some of my own speculations related to an evolutionary view of the human family and brain. While I have been interested in evolutionary biology for a number of decades, I am not a biologist nor do I pretend to be an expert on evolutionary theory. Therefore, I ask the reader to take my own speculations with a grain of salt. Bowen theory is not based on these speculations. It is difficult, however, to be as engaged in the effort to understand human behavior, the family, and Bowen theory as I have been without having an interest in evolutionary biology and how it might account for a fuller understanding of the family as a natural system. And so the evolutionary speculations in this chapter are mine and not meant to convey they are the principal views of those with a Bowen theory perspective.

Another important element in gaining knowledge about evolution and thinking of the family and human behavior as a part of evolution is the contribution it makes to a greater understanding of the emotional system as it is conceptualized in Bowen theory. It is difficult to communicate how basic the emotional system is to all our thoughts, feelings, and behavior. In Bowen theory it refers to the basic processes of all life. It is represented in the expression of life's many forms which have evolved over the history of evolution. And the functioning of the human family is viewed as such an expression. The human is unique, however, in the potential for some choice in our behavior based on evolution's gift of our elaborate brains. The neuroscientist Joaquin Fuster describes this gift and its potential in writing:

> Something radically new, however, takes place in the human brain that is unprecedented in prior evolution. Largely on account of the extraordinary evolutionary growth of its prefrontal cortex, the human brain "opens" to the future. The cerebral cortex of the human has become predictive. With that change, selection can be made between *anticipated* options of percept and action to occur in the future. (Fuster, 2013)

From this perspective, the human not only has the potential to observe and be aware of our behavior but in addition has the capacity to have some choice in how we behave. We are able to assess the impact our automatic or thoughtful behavior will have and the potential to adjust our behavior based on such assessments.

Bowen theory posits that the family emotional system is central in shaping the developmental process. This would include the maturation or differentiation of the higher cortical systems involved in self-regulation and in choice. It is not surprising that the family and an individual's brain functioning are so interlinked given what I would see as their coevolution. Bowen theory also posits that the differentiation of the higher cortical systems, which includes what Bowen defined as the intellectual system, is related to the maturation of an individual "self." The development of an individual self occurs in the context of the family emotional system. As previously mentioned, variation in this developmental process involves the degree to which offspring and the parental family emotionally separate and the differentiation of the higher cortical systems involved in the functioning of the intellectual system.

Family in the broad sense can be seen as beginning prior to the emergence of mammals as some reptilian and even fish species evolved to engage in protective behaviors of their offspring after they were hatched. And there have even been some fish and reptilian species in which fathers played a protective role. But it was with the emergence of mammalian life that the family/brain coevolution took off. Parental care permitted a longer period of development for more complex brains, which in turn allowed offspring to learn more from the present environment and from the experience of the previous generation. For most mammalian species, but not all, maternal care is central following birth. Biological substrates evolved to insure the bonds necessary for the parent–offspring relationships required for the prolonged period of parental care necessary for the development of more complex brains (Carter, 2005).

The complex brains of primates, and other large-brained animals, are not found without a prolonged period of development and parental care. The increase in the complexity of the brain and intelligence did not evolve independently from the relationship environment in which it evolved. The remarkable evolution of the human brain, tripling in size in the last two million years, occurred in the context of an evolving family environment. This coevolutionary development can be seen as underlying the reciprocal influence between family functioning and brain development. The observation that variation within and between families in the degree to which this reciprocal influence affects the level of maturation attained by children, and their ability to utilize the intellectual system in managing self throughout the life course, is a central element in the family systems theory developed by Bowen.

The higher cortical systems of the neocortex and especially the prefrontal cortex (PFC) increased both in size and complexity over the course of hominin evolution. How the human brain expanded so rapidly in such a brief evolutionary period has been an active area of interest in evolutionary biology. What contributed to this rapid expansion and to the elaborate social cognitive abilities of the human which require such large and complex brains? The social environment has been viewed as central in this evolutionary development (Dunbar, 2016; Flinn, 2005).

For most of human evolution, the social environment consisted of large extended families and other unrelated members involving multiple caretakers of infants and a wide range of social interactions. Together, large extended families and large brains have been seen as central to the successful adaptation the human has come to occupy in a wide range of environments (Allman, 1999).

SOCIAL BRAIN HYPOTHESIS

Several hypotheses have been developed which relate to the family to account for the rapid expansion of the human brain. One is the social brain hypothesis developed, among others, by British anthropologist and evolutionary psychologist Robin Dunbar (2002; 2016). He writes,

> There is general consensus that the prime mover in primate brain evolution (and perhaps even that of all mammals and birds) is the evolution of more complex forms of sociality. . . In most mammals and birds, the social brain hypothesis appears as a relationship between brain size and the mating system, with monogamously pairbonded species having significantly larger brains than species that mate polygamously or promiscuously, and especially so if monogamy involves lifelong pairbonds. We think this is probably because longlasting pairbonds are cognitively much more demanding than the more casual relationships of species that mate promiscuously. (Dunbar, 2016 p. 59-60)

In a test of his hypothesis, Dunbar did a comparative study (Dunbar, 2002), positing that there would be a relationship between the size of the neocortex in relation to the rest of the brain and the group living size of primate species. He found such a correlation and then posited that given the human brain, 150 would be the number of individuals one could maintain a stable relationship with. This would be about the size of many large four generational extended families or clans which existed for much of our species' history (see figure 5.1).

And it is not only the size of the group but the behavioral complexity involved in the group which is related to variation in neocortex size among primates. In the rapidly evolving neocortex found in the hominin line, the greatest expansion occurred in the PFC. Given the size, complexity, and interdependence found in the social groups of hominins, it is suggested that there would be selective pressure for individual emotional self-regulation, involving the capacity to inhibit impulsive responses which might be detrimental to group cohesion, allowing individuals to function with greater tolerance and cooperation.

The social brain hypothesis appears to be supported by observations of extant hunter-gatherer societies according to Dunbar. They have been found to live in multilevel forms of social organization. Dunbar describes this range in size:

> In hunter-gatherers, these (levels) consist of families, camp groups (or bands), communities (or clans), endogamous communities (or mega-bands), and ethnolinguistic units (or tribes. (Dunbar, 2016 p. 67)

The Social Cortex

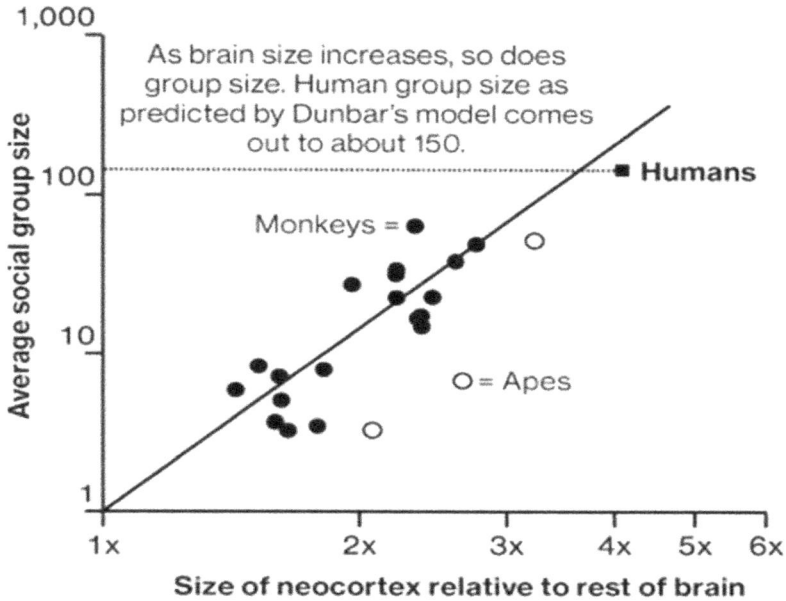

As brain size increases, so does group size. Human group size as predicted by Dunbar's model comes out to about 150.

DATA: THE SOCIAL BRAIN HYPOTHESIS, DUNBAR 1998

Figure 5.1   Relationship of Brain and Group Size. © Dunbar, 1988. Reproduced with permission.

He goes on to describe that the social complexity of the communities or clans consisting of about 150 as opposed to the larger groups in which the clan or community is nested:

Those within are people we know as individuals, based on relationships that have historical depth and involve trust, obligation and reciprocity; they are the people that we don't really think twice about helping when they ask. (Dunbar, 2016 p. 77)

Dunbar (2016) cites a number of historical and current human groups in which their typical size are in line with this hypothesis:

• Neolithic villages in the Middle East (6500–5500 BC) with a typical size of 150–200.
• Average county village (1085 AD) 150.
• Eighteenth-century English villages with a mean size of 160.

- Hunter-gatherer societies having a mean clan size of 165.
- East Tennessee rural mountain communities 197.

The social brain hypothesis suggests that the dramatic expansion of the neocortex, and especially the PFC, was selected for due to the advantage it provided individuals in adapting to the social complexity evolving in the hominin line. Dunbar suggests that two major revolutions occurred about 12,000 to 8,000 years ago: the living together in fixed settlements and the development of agriculture. While agriculture is often believed to be central in the emergence of larger communities, Dunbar holds that the real revolution occurred in the ability to live in fixed settlements. In order for this to occur, Homo sapiens had to develop a way to manage the social stresses which occur in such environments. An important function of the human PFC, of course, allowed the human to inhibit emotionally reactive behaviors which are disruptive in the more complex and integrated living systems. The living together in fixed settlements required the human to adapt to a new level of social complexity and successful adaptation required a new level of self-regulation in this new social environment.

SOCIAL SELECTION HYPOTHESIS

A related hypothesis which attempts to account for the rapid expansion of the brain found in Homo sapiens has been developed by Richard Alexander, an evolutionary biologist at the University of Michigan. He described a suite of characteristics which are unique to the human (Alexander, 1990; Flinn, Geary, & Ward, 2005). Among the characteristics found in large clans are

- extensive bi-parental care
- physically altricial infants
- prolonged childhood
- pair-bonded mating in multi-male groups
- concealed ovulation
- menopause
- large brains
- complex social groups
- linguistic and social learning aptitudes.

Some of these characteristics are found in other species, but the human is unique in having all of them. The complex social environment evolving in the hominin line created what they describe as a social selection pressure for intelligence.

Darwin distinguished between natural and social selection in that the latter refers to the selection of traits which result from competition among members of the same species (Flinn & Alexander, 2007). Within group competition is posited as leading to the selection of characteristics favorable to enhanced social competencies. The social environment appears to have become a primary selective pressure for the human and a family environment which includes care and social experience from both fathers and mothers as well as siblings and grandparents greatly contributed to the development of social competencies for the child.

The prolonged period of parental and alloparental care permitted the infant/ child/adolescent to develop in a protective environment and provided the context for the developing brain to learn and adapt to a complex and ever-changing social environment (Flinn, 2006). It allowed for the acquisition of language and knowledge required for social competency in the larger social arena.

The social and not the physical environment became the foremost adaptive challenge for the human, leading to a competitive "arms race" selecting for greater intelligence. The selective pressure for the expansion of the human brain, is posited as having occurred in the context of an evolving family environment (Flinn, Quinlan, Coe, & Ward, 2007). The task of managing self in more complex and highly integrated social units favored the selection of neural systems which could more accurately assess the behavior and intentions of others (theory of mind) and regulate the reflexive emotional responses of self to the context at hand. As Allman (1999) writes, "the development of the brain to the level of complexity we enjoy—and that makes our lives so rich—depended on the establishment of the human family as a social and reproductive unit." (p. 2) According to the social selection hypothesis, the complexity of the social environment was central in the selection of this complex brain of ours.

COOPERATIVE BREEDING HYPOTHESIS

Another hypothesis attempting to account for the rapid enlargement of the human brain and its exceptional cognitive abilities is referred to as the cooperative breeding hypothesis, first introduced by anthropologist and primatologist Sarah Hrdy (1999). It is based on those species in which parental care involves others in the social group beyond the mother. It may include fathers, siblings, grandmothers, and others. This hypothesis, supported by a large comparative study of primate species (Burkart, Hrdy, & Van Schaik, 2009), posits that though prolonged parental care and development is found among the great apes, the human is the only great ape to engage in cooperative breeding. The other great apes such as orangutans, gorillas, and chimpanzees are characterized by exclusive maternal care, with minimal involvement in infant caretaking by others.

Although rare among primates, cooperative breeding is found among some of the New World monkeys such as marmosets and tamarins (Snowdon & Ziegler, 2007). While they do not have large neocortices, they have been found to have socio-cognitive skills superior to their sister taxa, such as capuchin and squirrel monkeys, which do not engage in cooperative breeding. Cooperative breeders were found to have socio-cognitive skills such as "attentional biases toward monitoring others, the ability to coordinate actions spatially and temporally, increased social tolerance, increased responsiveness to others' signals, and spontaneous prosociality" (Burkart & van Schaik 2010, p.1). They hypothesize that the addition of the increased social cognitive abilities found in cooperative breeding species to the already extraordinary cognitive capacities found among the great apes resulted in the expanded human brain with its advanced socio-cognitive skills. They write,

> In sum, in nonhuman primates, canids, and elephants, cooperative breeding is associated not only with increased levels of social tolerance and responsiveness to the signals and needs of others, but also with the presence of spontaneous pro-social motivations, which extend beyond infants and sometimes beyond food to information, resulting in teaching. (Burkart, Hrdy, & Van Schaik, 2009 p. 180)

Other primates and the other great apes demonstrate social tolerance toward others, but it is the expression of proactive prosociality which is seen as underlying what has been described as human "hyper-cooperation" (Burkart et al., 2014). The other great apes demonstrate what is called "reactive prosociality," that is, individuals will respond to the signals of need by others but do not do so spontaneously. It is the "hyper-cooperation" found in the human which is posited as contributing to the emergence of human culture. In a prosociality study consisting of 24 groups of 15 primate species, Burkart et al. (2014) found that cooperative breeding was the best predictor of proactive prosociality among the various primate species. Other cooperative breeding primate species, such as the callitrichids (tamarins and marmosets), were found to exhibit proactive sociality in which they spontaneously would assist others in the group, but this characteristic was not found among our closest primate relatives, the great apes.

An additional socio-cognitive skill found among cooperative breeders is that of shared intentionality, which involves the capacity to engage with others in shared goals and intentions. This skill is absent in the other great apes and involves understanding others, an increased ability to communicate coopera-tive intentions, and collaborating in the pursuit of goals. Shared intentionality also includes the capacity for social and instructed learning (Burkart, Hrdy, & Van Schaik, 2009). In chimpanzees, for example, the young can learn skills from adults, such as using grass as a tool in the capturing of termites, though there is some question whether the adults are intentionally teaching the young chimps. In cooperative breeding species, however, such intentional teaching can be found. Along with "hyper-cooperativity," shared intentionality can be seen as a socio-cognitive skill not found among the other great apes. Psychologist Michael Tomasello describes this skill in writing:

> Conceiving of "I" and "you" as equivalent partners within our cooperative "we"—that is, conceiving of one another as cooperative second-personal agents—characterizes everything from dividing the spoils of a collaborative effort fairly among participants to citizens debating with one another in a modern civil society. Again, this is precisely those sociocultural activities that other great apes can neither create nor understand. (Tomasello, 2019 p. 312)

EXPENSIVE BRAIN HYPOTHESIS

Another related hypothesis relevant to the coevolution of the family and brain is the expensive brain hypothesis. Large brains are nutritionally expensive, especially early in development, with infants spending up to 60 percent of their resting metabolism on the brain and adults up to 25 percent. John Allman (1999) raises some of the questions related to how such an expensive biological system could evolve in writing:

> Animals with big brains are rare. If brains enable animals to adapt to changing environments, why is it that so few animals have large brains? The reason is that big brains are very expensive, costly in terms of time, energy, and anatomical complexity. Large brains take a long time to mature, and consequently large-brained animals are dependent on their parents for a long time. The slow development of large-brained offspring and the extra energy required to support them reduce the reproductive potential of the parents. . . . The basic question is, how do those few animals with large brains bear these extra costs? (p. 160)

Humans not only have larger brains than the other great apes but have a higher reproductive output as well. The energy cost of providing the nutrition and care for the large-brained human requires more than a mother alone can provide. For Homo sapiens, the mother–infant relationship depended on others to provide significant levels of alloparental care (Hrdy 2005). Clans or extended kin networks became central for development, influencing both caretaking and the developing brain.

In a comparative study of 478 mammal species, it was found that alloparental care contributes to a higher fertility rate among mammals, but only when it included paternal care was it related to the evolution of larger brains (Heldstab, Isler, Burkart, & Carels, 2019). The hypothesis presented is that while alloparental care provided by siblings or other family members contributes to the energy demands of child-care, such provision is not reliably stable over longer periods. During its prolonged period of growth, brain tissue develops at a constant rate and requires a consistent input of energy. In the species which are socially monogamous, the fathers were found to contribute a steadier nutritional contribution than those in which they were not involved in parental care. This combination is hypothesized to explain why humans differ from the other apes in having both an extremely large brain and a relatively high reproductive output.

All four of these hypotheses, I believe, contribute to a view that the coevolution of the family and the brain were central to the evolution of our species. The complete dependency of an infant on caretakers at birth, preceded by a prolonged gestational period and followed by future years of extended parental involvement over the course of development, is a vital element in the growth and development of both the brain and the individual. The increased integration of the family, along with the biological substrates involved in this integration, included monogamous mating pairs and a larger extended clan or family, principally grandmothers, older siblings, aunts, uncles, and so on.

Building on the maternal/offspring attachments of our mammalian ancestors to include biparental care and extended family alloparental care involved profound adaptations in the hominin biology (Flinn, Ward, and Noone 2005). Neuroendocrine processes regulating mother–infant involvement were expanded to other relationships to include the interdependent attachments observable in the human family. The complete dependency of an infant on caretakers at birth, followed by future years of extended parental care over the course of development, involves more than the mother–infant dyad (Donley, 2016). The increase in responsiveness among family members increased the influence the family unit had on development and the functioning of its members which includes not only their higher cortical systems but the other neuroendocrine systems as well. The neuroendocrine substrates linking individuals in lengthy attachments among the family's multiple members were an integral part of the evolving brain (Carter 2005) among humans and other primates (Storey & Ziegler 2015).

One of the shifts in the neuroendocrine substrates that occurred in the evolution from small-brained to large-brained animals found among primates involved the "social glue" underlying social bonding. Among smaller-brained mammals, the social glue involved the neuropeptides oxytocin and vasopressin which were involved in parental–offspring bonds. These neuropeptides were activated through olfactory processing. Due to the energetic costs of larger brains, primates required parental care beyond that of the mother. The social glue holding the larger social groups together found among primates, such as baboons and chimpanzees, required a transition from the brain's olfactory processing of oxytocin and vasopressin to complex visual processing (Curley & Keverne, 2005). Primates now maintained their social bonds through social interactions such as grooming which releases endorphins (Dunbar, 2016). The selection for increased social group size and alloparental care included biological substrates and greater complexity of interactions. These evolutionary developments both provided selective pressure for larger brains and were required to sustain them. In discussing the social bonds of larger-brained primates, James Curley and Eric Keverne (2005) write,

> Parenting and alloparenting are lifetime occupations for females in the group, an evolutionary development that has had a profound impact on brain evolution. Brain growth is energetically costly and postponing the greater part of this to the postpartum period has not only conserved the energetic demands of pregnancy on mother but has also ensured that the brain develops in an environment that facilitates the social learning that becomes integral to achieving adult bonding. (p. 565)

The family and the development of the brain have been inextricably woven together over the course of hominin evolution and are central to the capacity of individuals to successfully navigate through the social complexity of human life. This coevolutionary development can be seen as underlying the reciprocal influence between family functioning and brain development. The family/brain coevolution, involving prolonged attachments and an increased capacity to self-regulate, along with an ability to accurately assess the intentions of others and engage in "hyper-cooperative" behaviors, may well have provided the foundation for larger communities and an expanded cultural evolution.

THE FAMILY AS A HIGHER LEVEL OF BIOLOGICAL ORGANIZATION

The rapid and extensive expansion of the neocortex found in the evolutionary line leading to Homo sapiens has been an active area of interest in evolutionary biology. This has included speculation about the role of the social context. Along with the brain, the evolution of the human family has also been a remarkable evolutionary development. Over the course of hominin evolution, the increased interdependence of individuals into the family system, involving an increased responsiveness and emotional involvement among its members, entailed an increase in the degree of coregulation occurring among its members. Although a significant level of coregulation in the functioning of individuals in other primate groups has been found, it does not appear to be close to level of integration found in the human family. And while the human family exhibits such a high level of interdependence, the selection for the higher cortical systems found in the human also allowed for an increase in the capacity to self-regulate in the mid of this connectedness.

It is interesting to speculate as to the extent to which the integration and coregulation observable in the human family resulted in the evolution of a new biological whole. The emergence of increasingly complex systems has been central in the evolution of life. As evolutionary biologist Jan Sapp (2003) writes,

> evolution is a process of integration as well as divergence; there is divergence in the production of new life forms, but there is integration when these entities unite so as to make new wholes. These unions are recognized to be at the basis of the major transformations in the evolution of life: the origin of cells, organelles, and multicellular organisms. (p. 252)

Did the coevolution of the family and the brain lead to a reproductive unit operating at a new level of complexity—a unit which became the foundation for larger social and cultural systems? Living systems can vary in the level of their integration and the degree to which regulatory processes are centralized. Such processes are generally bidirectional and the components reciprocally influential. Biologist Deborah Gordon's (2010) study of ant colonies provides an example of a higher-level unit regulating the functioning of its members and how much remains to be learned about the functioning of such complex systems. She writes,

> The patterns or regularities in ant colony behavior are produced by networks of interaction among ants. The networks of interaction are complicated, irregular, noisy, and dynamic. The network is not a hidden program or set of instructions. There is no program—that's what is mind-boggling, and perhaps it is why at the beginning of the twenty-first century, there is so much we do not understand about biology. (Gordon, 2010 p. 47)

To date, the discussion of the family as a higher level of complexity, involved in the regulation of its members, has been largely absent in the sciences. Family is generally described as a social group or collection of individuals, overlooking its functioning as a distinct biological entity. Family is often viewed as a social entity shaped by a gene-culture coevolutionary process (Henrich, 2020; Hill & Boyd, 2021). The diverse expressions of the human family, such as filial obligations, who can marry, intra- and inter-familial bonds, values and beliefs, and so on are shaped by cultural evolution. This of course is accurate, but from the perspective of Bowen theory there are deeper emotional processes inherent in the family as a natural system. As Papero writes,

> Often active below the threshold of a person's awareness, emotion involves multiple complex interactions of physiology and psychology that deeply influence the individual's functioning (how the individual responds to the conditions he or she faces). That functioning in turn unfolds in sets of reciprocal interactions with important others, each influencing the other to form repetitive sets or patterns. These patterns can be observed and predicted in conjunction with variables in context. (Papero, 2015 p. 15)

Culture influences how the family emotional system may be expressed such as involving social norms to be adhered to, but the underlying processes of the human family are viewed as based on biology and are universal. This proposition remains to be tested, but to date anecdotal observations appear to support it. It will be interesting to learn the extent to which the concepts in Bowen theory can be observed in all cultures. Is there a basic reproductive unit to which a number of individuals are attached? Does an emotional contagion observable in the transfer of anxiety among the members of a family exist? Can a level of fusion be observed in these units and are the adaptive mechanisms of distance, conflict, reciprocal functioning and the family projection process evident? Can a multigenerational transmission process be observed which generates variation in the adaptive capacity of individuals over multiple generations? Does a continuum of adaptive capacity, as defined in the concept of differentiation of self exist?

Whether the emergence of the human family represents a major evolutionary transition remains an open question, though some of the hypotheses related to the transition from single-celled to multicellular organisms can be applied (Libby & Rainey, 2013). The rapid expansion of the human brain has clearly been a factor in the rapid expansion of Homo sapiens. The emergence and ongoing evolution of culture is also central to the ecological dominance of the human. The emergence of the family as a reproductive unit represented a significant change from the reproductive systems found in our fellow great apes. Was the human family, in all of its culturally expressed forms, central to the development of the larger and more complex social and cultural systems which have occurred? The coevolution of the family and the brain would appear to be a plausible hypothesis as a central factor underlying the broader social developments leading to the dramatic growth and expansion of Homo sapiens. As neuroscientist John Allman wrote in his book *Evolving Brains* (1999), "The human evolutionary success story depends on two great buffers against misfortune, large brains and extended families, with each supporting and enhancing the adaptive value of the other" (p. 5).

Did this "success story" represent a major transformation in evolution? Did hominin evolution result in more than an extension of primate evolution, but in a transformation analogous to the emergence of nucleated cells or multicellular organisms? Did the coevolution of the family and the brain results in the emergence of an adaptive system at a new level of complexity? Did it provide the basis for the development of all those characteristics which have fueled the hype-cooperative, complex relationship systems found in the human? It is beyond my pay grade to engage in such lofty speculation, but I remain curious about what I would consider to be the observational blindness related to the central role the family plays in the human's adaptive capacity and in the leap in organizational complexity that occurred in this primate's evolution.

The evolutionary line leading to Homo sapiens diverged from the line of the modern chimpanzee line about six million years ago. A number of hominin lines evolved with Homo erectus being the most long lasting and living for almost 1.8 million years (Dunbar, 2016). During this period the brain showed only a small growth in its size. Dunbar describes brain growth occurring with the emergence of new hominin species. The expansion of the brain in these species occurred early in their evolution and remained stable throughout their existence. But about 500,000 years ago there occurred a dramatic growth in brain size among the first archaic humans, Homo heidelbergensis. Further growth in brain size occurred with the emergence of Homo sapiens only 200,000 years later. Dunbar (2016) writes,

> What produced this new development is not clear. Conventional wisdom points to climate change as the main driver of speciation (the process whereby new species emerge out of ancestral populations), and the origins of Homo sapiens may be no different. However, our species seems to have spread very quickly through Africa, quite rapidly replacing the archaic human populations. How and why they replaced archaics so quickly is rather a mystery, especially given the fact that archaics had successfully occupied Africa (and Europe) for at least 300,000 years by the time modern humans had appeared. (p. 15)

It is purely speculative on my part, but did the rapid brain growth during this period take place in relation to an increase in the integration of the family reproductive unit? Did competition between the newly emerged clans or tribes contribute to a selective pressure for the coevolution of larger brains and more integrated extended family systems? Did this evolutionary process involve the selection for the biological substrates underlying the increasingly interdependent attachments involved in the reproductive unit of the family? Did the accretion of small changes due to the selective advantages of a larger, more complex brain and a more integrated reproductive unit lead to a tipping point or phase shift, a new level of complexity and a transformative change in evolution? Did a more complex brain allow for a more complex relationship system and the more integrated relationship system of the family contribute to the selection for a more complex brain?

The study of cranial shape and size from the fossil record has allowed archeologists to determine brain growth over hominin evolution. Dunbar (2016) describes five major shifts or transitions occurring over hominin evolution from the Australopithecines to the modern human. Very rapid evolutionary change occurred during these transitions followed by long periods with little change. The last major transition occurred approximately 12,000 years ago when Homo sapiens transitioned from life as hunter-gatherers to living in fixed settlements. This appears to have been a self-protective development. There is fossil evidence of violence among various groups as 15 percent of deaths were due to warfare or some other form of violence (Dunbar, 2016). The death rate of 15 percent from violence among hunter-gatherers is similar to that found among current hunter-gatherer groups (Pinker, 2011). The transition to living in fixed settlements is not associated with significant changes in brain size but in their social groupings. The major challenge during this period had to do with managing the social stresses involved in living in larger groups.

Genetics of course were involved in the evolutionary developments along the hominin line. As mentioned earlier, recent knowledge about the structure and functioning of genes has led to the view that the genome is more plastic than originally thought. The interactions between genes and the environment is now known to be more active and reciprocally influential (Cole, 2013; Meaney, 2010). It has recently been suggested that the architecture of the genome and social behavior can coevolve. Rubenstein et al. (2019) write,

> Most studies examining the genomic underpinnings of social behavior are typically unidirectional, in that they seek to identify genes that underlie behavior, but fail to consider how social behavior might affect genome structure and function and thereby influence the evolution of the genome itself. Importantly, the genome is not simply a sequence of nucleotides or a collection of genes. Rather, the genome has an intricate architecture, including a complex regulatory machinery, mobile elements, and chemical modifications, all of which potentially influence—and can be influenced by—behavioral phenotypes in underappreciated ways. (p. 844)

To what extent might the convergent evolution of cooperative breeding and the large brains of the great apes have contributed to a change in the genomic architecture underlying the larger and more complex brains of Homo sapiens?

This proposal may be speculative at this point but it suggests another element that may have contributed to the rapid expansion of the human brain and support a family/brain coevolution hypothesis.

Did such a development lay the groundwork for the emergence of human culture, leading to the emergence of phenomena such as theory of mind, shared intentionality, and the hyper-cooperativity found in Homo sapiens? Homo sapiens emerged about 300,000 years ago, while a marked shift in the development of human culture looks to have occurred about only about 50,000 years ago. Did the family provide a building block for the emergence of larger communities? Natural communities of 150 have been found to consist of smaller subunits of 5, 15, and 50 individuals and extend to larger groupings of 500 and 1,500. Dunbar (2016) writes,

> The substructuring of primate groups owes its origins to the need to create coalitions or alliances that protect individuals against the costs of living in large groups. In effect, each layer provides the framework that supports the layer above, with the next layer being an emergent property of the layer below with the two held together in a complex tension. The substructuring of human communities will have arisen for the same reasons: at each level, the smaller grouping makes the existence of the next layer possible. (p. 292-293)

Did the emergence of the family provide the foundation for the larger layers leading to larger and more complex social groupings and the rapid expansion of culture? Dunbar further writes,

> The story of human evolution has been one of finding ways to adjust to that pressure (i.e. the need for defence against conspecific raiding) through novel solutions to the problems of social bonding and the nutrient demands of large bodies and brains. . . . But in the end, what has made us who we are has been a complex series of adjustments to the basic hominin physiological, social and cognitive design. It has, of course, been the cognitive changes that have given us the modern world of science and the arts, but it is the three together that have given us the rich tapestry of modern human relationships. (p. 344)

A core assumption of the theory developed by Murray Bowen is that the human family is a natural system and a product of evolution. As I mentioned earlier, however, it is a theory about how the family functions and not how it evolved. A view of the human family which functions as a biological system, has evolved over millions of years, and is central to the development and functioning of individuals, does however provide a different vantage point for the study of human behavior. As Michael Kerr (2019) posits,

Current evolutionary theory explains how variation in adaptive functioning evolves among species. Bowen theory explains how individual and family variation in the capacity for adaptation to life challenges evolves within the human species. (p. 119)

Bowen theory describes the role of the family in shaping the adaptive capacity of individuals and families. It does not seem to be too far out to posit that the evolution of the family might be intricately related to the rapid development of the brain and the emergence of the remarkable adaptive capacity of the human. In the next chapter, I will discuss the impact of life challenges on families and their adaptive capacity from the perspective of Bowen theory.

Chapter 6

The Impact of Stress on the Family and Adaptive Capacity

On September 18, 2017, the remote village of Bwa Mawego in the small eastern Caribbean island of Dominica experienced a direct hit by the hurricane Maria. As it approached the island it had been categorized as a category 3 tropical storm. The intensity of Maria climbed quickly, however, and by the time it made landfall at Bwa Mawego, on the rugged east coast of Dominica, it had reached a 5+ category, the highest possible rating.

The winds began to pick up about 5 p.m. and by 8 p.m., the wind and rain had reached their full level of intensity. With the exception of a brief interlude, as the eye of the hurricane passed over, Maria continued until 5 a.m. Winds of speed 175+ miles per hour and rain totaling 18 inches battered the village throughout the night. The destructiveness of the storm destroyed most of the village: its homes and vegetation flattened. Roads to Bwa Mawego were closed for weeks due to landslides and fallen trees. A helicopter passing over the village the morning after Maria reported that all of the village's residents had been lost. The village residents themselves feared other family members had been lost. Remarkably, all of the village's almost 400 inhabitants had survived. A tremendous relief was experienced when the hurricane passed, and families discovered that their other family members had survived. The impact of the hurricane, however, was significant and obviously continued into the months and several years which followed.

During the hurricane, families huddled in their homes or in a few of the homes in the village thought to be more structurally solid. In addition to the trauma experienced during the hurricane, families were faced with the full or partial destruction of their homes, food shortage, destruction of electrical and piped water systems, and for several weeks cutoff from communication with family members living off-island.

Bwa Mawego has been the site of a three-decade longitudinal study, led by anthropologist Mark Flinn of Baylor University. The study has included the collection of physiological and behavioral data related to the impact of stress on the health of the residents of this village (Flinn & England, 1998; Flinn, Ponzi, Nepomnaschy, & Noone, 2012). This ongoing and in-depth study has provided a rich view of the daily life of children and their families. In addition to twice weekly surveys of the children's health and family relationships, Flinn has collected cortisol, immunoglobulin, and other biological data on the village's children. His study has demonstrated the importance of family life on the health and behavior of children. Flinn's longitudinal study has been based on both a multigenerational and evolutionary perspective (Flinn, 2005; 2006).

In addition to providing humanitarian assistance in the year following Maria, Flinn and colleagues also collected markers of health and biological change. The analysis of pre- and post-hurricane changes has been undertaken, but an initial survey found that the death rate in the village increased from 4.6 deaths per year to 14 and a majority of the residents lost 5–10 percent of their body weight (Flinn, personal communication).

Hurricane Maria represented a natural disaster inflicting both immediate and ongoing damage to Bwa Mawego and its residents. From a Bowen theory perspective, individuals and families are generally able to cope with immediate threats in an effective manner. People can "rise to the occasion" and often function at higher levels during periods of intense stress. There is some evidence that a majority of people experience some trauma in their lives and are able to respond with some resilience (Bonanno, 2004). In my interviews of twenty-three mothers, two-and-a-half years after Maria regarding their experiences during and after the hurricane, I was impressed with their resilience and the resilience of the community. It was a traumatic experience that was shared by all. Despite a significant level of devastation, the village's residents have been recovering, though with varying degrees.

Individuals and families vary in their adaptive capacity and the degree to which stressful events will impact their physical, psychological, and social functioning. While all of Bwa Mawego's residents were subjected to the intensity and destructiveness of Maria, there was variation among individuals and families in how they recovered. Some people had sturdier homes which held up through the night. The location of homes varied in their vulnerability to the winds and rain. Some families had more provisions available to them in the days and weeks that followed the hurricane. In addition to these and other such variables, Bowen theory would posit there are three principal factors influencing the variation found in how adaptive people are in effectively responding to stress. These are (1) the level of differentiation of self (their basic level of adaptive capacity); (2) the level of chronic anxiety (level of extant allostatic load); and (3) the degree of isolation in an individual's or family's life. A fourth variable, which is related to the level of chronic anxiety, is how prolonged the stress persists (Gianaros et al., 2007; McEwen & Gianaros, 2011; Miller et al., 2009).

Individuals vary in their vulnerability to stress and gains have been made at the genetic (Cole, 2013: Ellis et al. 2011), epigenetic (McGowan, 2014; Meaney, 2010; Szyf, McGowan & Meaney, 2008), developmental (Barrett& Fleming, 2011; Gunnar 2005; Shonkoff et al., 2009), and social (Boyce & Kobor, 2015; McEwen & Gianaros 2010) levels in understanding factors contributing to differences in vulnerability or resilience among individuals in responding to life stressors. In a given population, the impact of an identical stressor will vary significantly in terms of its impact and how well people adapt to it. One factor in this variability is that of perception. Individuals vary in their ability to accurately distinguish between what is a clear and present threat and what is not. Those individuals less capable of making this distinction will maintain a greater level of wariness regarding potential threats, resulting in higher levels of chronic anxiety or allostatic load. George Slavich and Steven Cole point out the profound effect perception, as opposed to the reality of a situation, can have on triggering biological responses even to the extent of the expression of genes.

> The paramount role of subjective perception in human social signal transduction stems from the fact that central nervous system–mediated experiences of social-environmental conditions, not the external conditions themselves, are what trigger the release of neural and endocrine response molecules that proximally regulate gene expression. (Slavich & Cole, 2013)

Another factor contributing to the variation among individuals in how effectively they might respond to stress, of course, is the available resources at hand in responding to life challenges. The duration and severity of stress an individual experiences are also factors contributing to the development of symptoms. An individual might respond in a highly effective manner to a stressful event during a less challenging time in life but become symptomatic in responding to the same event during a period of prolonged or multiple life stress events.

At the individual level, the neuroendocrine stress response systems, the hypothalamic–pituitary–adrenal system (HPA) and the autonomic nervous system (ANS), along with the immune system, have been selected for over the course of evolution to allow organisms to respond to environmental and internal threats (McEwen, 2007). Largely automatic, they trigger physiological and behavioral responses designed to enable an individual to marshal the energy required for the "fight, flight, or freeze" responses necessary for

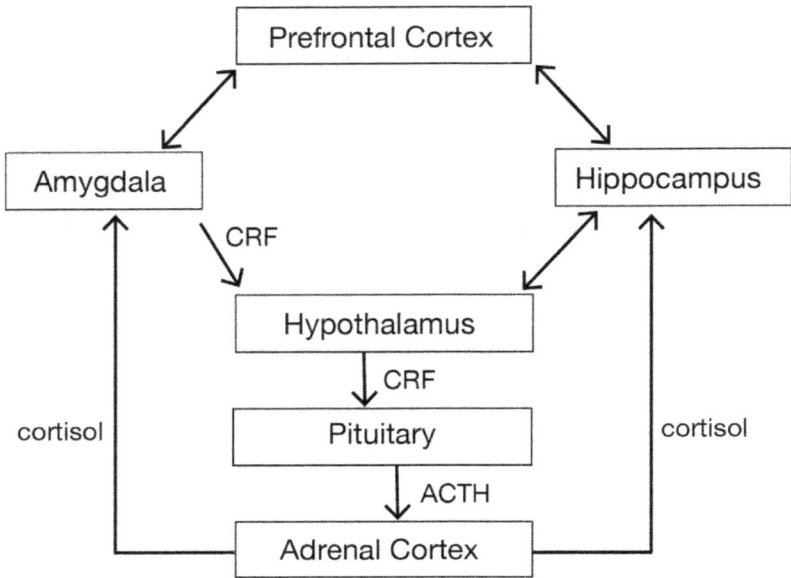

Figure 6.1 The Hypothalamic–Pituitary–Adrenal Stress Response System. *Source:* Created by the author.

survival. The threats may be due to a serious physical injury, a natural disaster, or social in nature. Given that our emotional well-being is so intimately connected to our important relationships, a disturbance such as a significant loss or threatened loss to a loved one will also have a physiological response (Eisenberger, 2011).

A brief description of the HPA system provides an example of the integration of regulatory systems involved in an individual's response to stress (see figure 6.1). When a perception of threat occurs, the amygdala releases corticotropin releasing factor (CRF) which is picked up by receptors on the hypothalamus, signaling it to secrete CRF to the pituitary gland. The pituitary gland then releases the stress hormone adrenocorticotropic hormone (ACTH) into the bloodstream and which is then picked up by receptors on the cortex of the adrenal gland inducing it to release the stress hormone cortisol into the bloodstream. In traveling through the bloodstream, cortisol signals the various regulatory systems (cardiovascular, respiratory, immune, digestive, and reproductive systems) to effectively respond to the challenge.

In a feedback loop, cortisol is later picked up by receptors in the brain. This process plays an important role in regulating the HPA system. For when cortisol levels are elevated for prolonged periods, they can result in a dysregulation in one or more of the physiological systems involved. The hippocampus plays an important function in this process. When cortisol is picked up by hippocampal receptors, it then signals the hypothalamus to decrease its release of CRF, ending the HPA stress response system. In a counterbalancing process, cortisol also feeds back to the amygdala signaling it to continue releasing CRF.

The prefrontal cortex (PFC), rich in cortisol receptors, is also involved. Through its neural connections with the amygdala, it has the capacity to put the brakes on the HPA system. The PFC and the hippocampus are the principal brain structures involved in inhibiting the cortisol stress response. The prolonged elevation of cortisol, however, can result in the loss of the hippocampal and PFC's effectiveness in regulating the response to stress, thus increasing the potential for symptom development. While there is a good deal of variability involving other factors, prolonged and severe stress in the family early in life may impact the effectiveness of the stress response systems of children throughout the life course (Anacker et al., 2014; Essex et al. 2002).

Stress, of course, is inherent to life as individuals adapt to their physical and social environments. When the response to stress is effective, such adaptiveness can contribute to an individual's well-being and enhance their ability to adapt to future challenges they may encounter. On the other hand, when stress exceeds an individual's capacity to effectively respond for a prolonged period, it can adversely affect their health.

A wealth of research evidence over the past several decades supports the relationship between stressful life events and health. This evidence has contributed to an understanding of how stress and the response of individuals to stress are significant factors in the development of physical, emotional, and behavioral symptoms. Knowledge about the neuroendocrine systems involved in the physiological stress response and their influence on various other systems has shed light on how the response to stress can contribute to a wide range of health problems (McEwen, 2007; McEwen & Gianaros, 2010; Miller, Rohleder & Cole, 2009). The observation of the family as an interdependent functioning system has contributed to an understanding of how a disturbance in the family relationship system can trigger the physiological stress response in individuals. Since emotionally important relationships are a principal element in people's well-being, a threat to one or more of those relationships is typically experienced as a threat to self.

The stress response systems are vital to our survival. They provide the necessary energy and activation of the physiological and behavioral responses required for effectively responding to life challenges. The higher cortical systems, such as the PFC, play an important role in effectively responding to stress and in regulating the stress response systems. They can, for example, allow one to distinguish between real versus imagined threats and thus serve to effectively regulate the more automatic physiological, emotional, and behavioral responses (McEwen, 2007; Silvers, 2013). The prospect of public speaking, for example, may trigger a substantial fear response for some. The higher cortical systems, however, can allow an individual to learn to override the fear response to a greater or lesser degree and allow him or her to accomplish a goal they have set for themselves.

The regulation of the stress response systems is particularly important as their inadequate or excessive activation can create significant emotional or physical health problems. A primary function for all living beings is to maintain a stable internal homeostasis in the face of a changing environment. When that homeostatic balance is disturbed or threatened, physiological mechanisms are activated by the brain to preserve the integrity of the organism. The term "allostasis," originally introduced by Peter Sterling (Sterling & Eyers, 1988), has been highlighted by Bruce McEwen (McEwen & Gianaros, 2011) to describe the adaptive mechanisms necessary for the maintenance of an individual's homeostasis.

ALLOSTASIS AND ALLOSTATIC LOAD

A key function of the brain is to monitor the body and the environment and to activate or inhibit the responses necessary in adapting to change. When someone begins to jog, for example, cardiac and pulmonary functions are called upon to meet the necessary blood and oxygen levels the major muscles require. After running, the physiological systems involved return to baseline. When a threat is perceived, the HPA and ANS neuroendocrine systems signal the various physiological and behavioral systems required to effectively respond. Following a wound, for example, proinflammatory immune cells are secreted from bone marrow to fight infection. This immune response is activated by the ANS (Miller, Rohleder, & Cole, 2009). The term "allostasis" refers to the processes triggered in response to challenge. The brain is involved in both triggering allostatic processes and in putting the brakes on them when they are no longer needed. Allostasis is vital in maintaining an individual's homeostasis. While it is essential that the stress response system mechanisms be activated in response to a threat, it is also important that they be inactivated as their prolonged activation leads to a wearing down of a number of neuroendocrine functions such as the cardiovascular and immune systems. The wearing down of the brain and body resulting from the over- or under-activation of allostatic mechanisms is referred to as allostatic load (McEwen & Gianaros, 2010). The prolonged activation of the immune system would be an example of an allostatic mechanism, which can result in allostatic load and then a host of symptoms.

The chronic activation of the stress response systems can result in the loss of effectiveness of brain regions such as the PFC, hippocampus, and amygdala, all of which play key roles in regulating the HPA and ANS systems. In addition to chronic stress, the elevated and chronic anticipation of real or perceived threats can also lead to conditions of allostatic load. Multiple factors can go into variation of the level of allostatic load an individual may carry. There is some evidence of genetic involvement which can contribute to an increased sensitivity to stress (Boyce & Ellis, 2005; Ellis et al., 2011). The shaping of heightened stress reactivity can also result from epigenetic processes occurring in utero and throughout the course of development (Anacker, et al., 2014; Champagne, 2008; Lupien et al., 2009). Central to all the factors related to the development of allostatic load, including the genetic, is the environment an individual lives in during the course of development. The family is the principal social environment during development and the concept of the family emotional system, as defined in Bowen theory, represents a conceptual framework for both understanding variation in the development of allostatic load and for integrating knowledge related to the impact of stress from the various scientific disciplines.

The consideration of early life adversity in the stress literature has largely been focused on abuse, neglect, and stressful environments. While the family is acknowledged as a principal environment influencing development, the study of the family and its influence on the development of resilience or vulnerability to an individual's health has to some degree been overlooked. Papero (2017) has reviewed a number of the studies looking at the impact of major stressors on families, but the view of the family as an adaptive system involved in regulating the physiological as well as the psychological functioning of its members has not been widely studied.

CHRONIC ANXIETY AND THE FAMILY

Bowen theory posits that the adaptive capacity of individuals is principally influenced by one's level of differentiation and the level of chronic anxiety. In describing the relationship between differentiation of self and chronic anxiety, Kerr (Kerr & Bowen, 1988) writes,

> The higher the level of chronic anxiety in a relationship system, the greater the strain on people's adaptive capabilities. Adaptiveness has been exceeded when the intensity of a person's anxious response to stress impairs his own functioning and/or the functioning of those with whom he is emotionally connected. The functional impairment can range from mild to serious physical, emotional, or social symptoms. Symptom development, therefore, depends on the amount of stress *and* on the adaptiveness of the individual or family to stress. Highly adaptive people and families require considerable stress to trigger symptoms.

Poorly adaptive people and families can be symptom free if the level of chronic anxiety is low. (Kerr & Bowen, 1988 p.112)

Chronic anxiety is distinguished from acute anxiety in that the latter represents a response to a real and current threat. In general, people adapt well to the immediate challenges they are faced with. The loss of a job, a divorce, or a natural disaster, such as the experience of hurricane Maria that the residents of Bwa Mawego experienced, are major stressors for individuals and families. The effects of time-limited stressors may continue for some time, but there is usually an awareness of what needs to be done in response to them. Traumatic events may test the resilience of people, but most recover over a period of time (Bonanno, 2004).

Chronic anxiety represents more of a fear about what might happen. All people maintain a certain level of chronic anxiety varying only in degree. Mark Twain was quoted as saying something to the effect of "I've lived through many tragedies in my life, some of which actually happened." How often have you found yourself worrying about some future event only to recognize your worry was unfounded once the event has occurred or perhaps never occurred.

Heightened chronic anxiety can operate as a general wariness and involve the stress response systems even when it is operating outside of our awareness. It can take the form of worry about one's health or that of important others. For some it may consist of a concern about finances even when by all objective appearances their financial status is quite secure. When sufficiently heightened, chronic anxiety can result in a level of allostatic load and the development of physical, psychiatric, or behavioral symptoms.

Joseph LeDoux distinguishes between fear and anxiety in a manner similar to how acute and chronic anxiety are defined in Bowen theory. LeDoux (2015) writes,

Somewhat different brain mechanisms are engaged when the state is triggered by an objective and present threat as opposed to an uncertain event that may or may not occur in the future. An immediately present stimulus that is itself dangerous, or that is a reliable indicator that danger is likely to soon follow, results in fear. . . . However, when the state in question involves worry about something that is not present and may never occur, then the state is anxiety. (pp. 10–11)

The level of differentiation of self generally determines the range of chronic anxiety an individual experiences. Differentiation remains quite stable throughout adulthood, while one's level of chronic anxiety fluctuates based on the level of stress an individual and family may be experiencing. But two families experiencing similarly prolonged stressful events will exhibit different levels of chronic anxiety based on their levels of differentiation. The degree of differentiation of the higher cortical systems, defined in the theory as the intellectual system, determines to what extent an individual is capable of regulating the emotional system, which includes the stress response systems. Under sufficient stress, the higher cortical systems are overridden by the subcortical systems involved in the stress response systems (Arsten, 2009; Arnsten, Wang, & Paspalas, 2012). In describing the influence of subcortical systems on the functioning of the PFC during stress, Yale University neuroscientist Amy Arnsten writes,

> Under conditions of psychological stress the amygdala activates stress pathways in the hypothalamus and brainstem, which evokes high levels of noradrenaline and dopamine release. This impairs PFC regulation but strengthens amygdala function, thus setting up a "vicious cycle." . . . Thus, attention regulation switches from thoughtful "top-down" control by the PFC that is based on what is most relevant to the task at hand to "bottom-up" control by the sensory cortices, whereby the salience of the stimulus (for example, whether it is brightly coloured, loud, or moving) captures our attention. . . . Thus, during stress, orchestration of the brain's response patterns switches from slow, thoughtful PFC regulation to the reflexive and rapid emotional responses of the amygdala and related subcortical structures. (Arnsten, 2009 p. 414)

Figure 6.2 depicts neural pathways influencing the functioning of the PFC. Two areas in the brainstem, the locus coeruleus (LC) and the ventral tegmental area (VTA), produce norepinephrine (NE) and dopamine (DA), which at moderate levels enhance the functioning of the PFC. With the perception of a threat, however, the amygdala signals the brainstem areas to increase the production of NE and DA. This has the dual effect of impairing PFC functioning and strengthening the fear response mediated by the amygdala. Again, as Arnsten writes,

> Thus, during stress, orchestration of the brain's response patterns switches from slow, thoughtful PFC regulation to the reflexive and rapid emotional responses of the amygdala and related subcortical structures. (Arnsten, 2009 p. 414)

This makes sense from an evolutionary perspective as the more automatic survival circuits occur earlier in development and in evolution and respond automatically to a perceived threat. While the brain's neural systems interact in a reciprocal manner, the earlier evolved systems involved in the stress response are dominant during stress (Panksepp 1998).

As previously mentioned, Bowen theory posits that over the course of development, individuals vary in the degree to which the functioning of

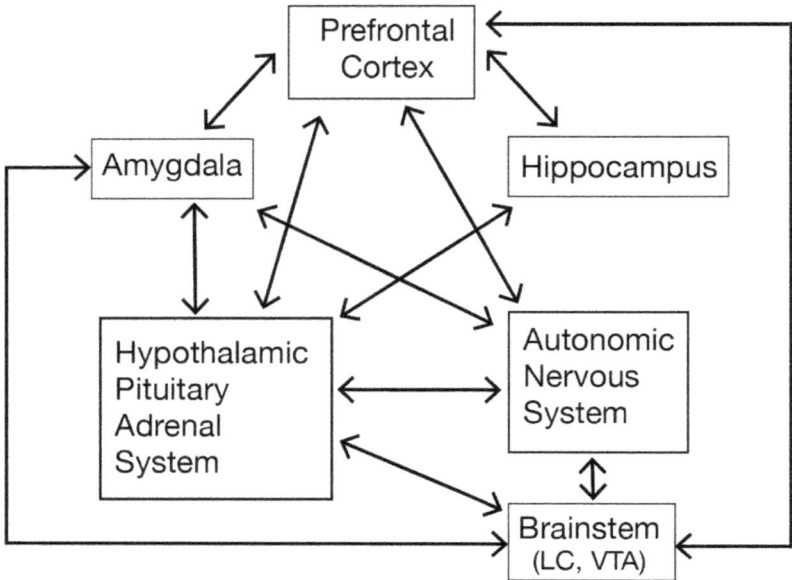

Figure 6.2   Influence of Brainstem Functioning on the PFC during Stress. *Source:* Created by the author.

higher cortical systems (intellectual system) develop. This development includes the function of distinguishing between thoughts and feelings (Bowen, 1978). Individuals differ in what they perceive to be stressful and in their ability to have some choice in how they respond to stress. And even though the emotional system may override the intellectual system during periods of significant stress, it will take a greater level of stress for this override to occur for individuals at higher levels of differentiation of self. A difference can also be found among individuals in their capacity to recover from intense or prolonged stressful events. The sudden and unexpected loss of a job, for example, may result in two individuals being overwhelmed by a fear of what the future will bring. Each may remain anxious or fearful about this new status, but the one with more adaptive capacity will begin to more realistically assess the situation earlier than one whose intellectual or thinking system remains submerged in fear.

Variation in the intermix of intellectual and emotional functioning, while influenced by the degree and length of stress, is viewed in Bowen theory as principally shaped by the relationship system of the family (Noone, 2016). Chronic anxiety is seen as a property of the family emotional system and its members. At greater levels of oneness or undifferentiation, family members are more sensitized to the functioning of each other and as a result their own functioning is more vulnerable to being regulated by family interactional processes than by themselves. An increase in anxiety by one family member will more easily transfer to an increase in the anxiety of others. At higher levels of differentiation, members have a greater capacity to regulate their own emotional functioning even when another member may have a spike in their level of anxiety.

It is important to note that all families have greater levels of oneness or undifferentiation than they are usually aware of. That individuals and families exist along a continuum of emotional interdependence is an evident aspect of the human phenomenon. The continuum of differentiation of self, posited by Bowen (1978), can be seen as a baseline for the level of chronic anxiety evidenced by families. The impact of stressful events will then vary among families based on where they exist on this continuum. Families at the lower end of the continuum of differentiation or adaptive capacity can be thought of as carrying more of an allostatic load. Their resourcefulness in the face of life's challenges is more constricted than those families carrying less of a load, less chronic anxiety.

At higher levels of chronic anxiety, the family adaptive mechanisms will become more exaggerated and utilized to a greater extent than they would for families at lower levels. There is a predictability about the utilization of these mechanisms by families, which is evident with a careful recording of the history of family events and family functioning. A family which principally utilizes the child projection process can be observed to increase their concern or focus on a child during stressful periods and that child will predictably respond. Families vary in the degree to which they utilize one mechanism or several, but it is predictable that one of the mechanisms will be triggered in response to an increase in chronic anxiety.

It is only when viewed at the family level of organization that the mechanisms can be seen as adaptive. The anxious focus on a child may appear maladaptive when symptoms develop for a child, but it can stabilize the family unit in response to its level of chronic anxiety. Tension in the marital pair, for example, may be stabilized by a common concern about a child. One individual described a significant level of conflict between him and his wife during the first five years of their marriage. When their first child was born, he said their conflict became minimal based on what he saw as their finding "a common cause." The child focus also represents an adaptive response by the child to the family unit. Though it may constrict the child's development to an extent in the long term, its stabilizing effect on the unit can be a functional response by the parents and child. Less anxious parents are a plus for the child in the short term.

Similar to the allostatic mechanisms described at the level of the individual by McEwen (2007), the family adaptive mechanisms, when over-utilized for prolonged periods, can result in a "wear and tear" on the family relationship processes and the development of chronic symptoms. Repetti et al. (2011) describe what can "reflect 'adaptive trade-offs' that balance short-term survival advantages under harsh rearing conditions against disadvantages manifested later in development" (p. 921). While a child focus can result from "harsh rearing conditions," it also is found in what would be considered "loving rearing conditions." It is not so much whether the parental overinvolvement is positive or negative, but the intensity or level of involvement that can be constricting. In an interesting study of fifty young adults, Narita et al. (2010), using neuroimaging, found that higher paternal and maternal overprotection during their first sixteen years of life, correlated with a reduction in gray matter in the dorsal lateral PFC. The assessment of overprotective parenting was based on the results of a self-report instrument, but the study was rare in that it was not solely focused on harsh or traumatic early childhood experiences. The concept of the family projection process in Bowen theory posits that a persistent focus on a child as a response to tension in the marital relationship can result in that child's developing less emotional autonomy and less of a capacity to self-regulate.

The assessment of an individual's and family's level of chronic anxiety is vital for the clinician. Families look and function very differently when the level of chronic anxiety is higher than when it is lower in a unit. A more realistic assessment of a family's adaptive capacity can be made when their functioning can be viewed over time and in relation to the intensity of the current challenges they are confronted with. Too often a diagnosis is assigned to an individual when he or she is functioning at their lowest level. A broader view of their functioning and that of the larger family can provide a more objective view of their basic adaptive capacity. An appreciation of when a family may have been going through a prolonged regression is also useful for the individuals and families who are attempting to make gains during stressful periods. Kerr (2019 pp. 65–88) describes the impact of emotional regression on a family's functioning. In defining regression he writes,

> I define *emotional regression* in Bowen theory in a specific way: If chronic anxiety escalates in a relationship system, the system becomes dominated by less thoughtful and more reactive ways of interacting that are older in an evolutionary sense than the advanced complex behaviors of a well-functioning relationship system. (p. 65)

This definition of emotional regression in a relationship system appears analogous to the description of brain functioning under stress described earlier.

In the assessment of a family's functioning, Bowen theory presents a number of factors which influence their adaptive capacity. As mentioned, principal among these factors are a family's level of differentiation and their level of chronic anxiety. Others include the extent to which they are in viable contact with the extended family, their position in the multigenerational family, and the length and severity of the stressors they have recently experienced. It is clinically important to assess these factors and to engage one or more members of the family in that assessment. The clinical application of Bowen theory is not a subject of this book, but a couple of quotes by Bowen (Kerr & Bowen, 1988) illustrate the effect one family member can have during the course of the therapy.

> Operationally, ideal family treatment begins when one can find a leader with the courage to define self, who is as invested in the welfare of the family as in self, who is neither angry nor dogmatic, whose energy goes to changing self rather than telling others what they should do, who can know and respect the multiple opinions of others, who can modify self in response to the strengths of the group, and who is not influenced by the irresponsible opinions of others. When one family member moves toward "differentiation," the family symptoms disappear. (pp. 342–343)

In another quote Bowen describes the process occurring when a family member undertakes this effort:

> The process can be illustrated by a family in the undifferentiated range. It was a leaderless group. Passive decisions were made to "get along with the others." Potential differences surfaced in the form of chronic emotional and physical illness. Family members began a constant process of blaming each other. Finally, a more differentiated leader began to emerge. Instead of blaming the other person, he focused on himself. He lived his own life by example, instead of blaming. He became important to everyone in the relationship system. The family symptoms settled down. After several weeks, the leader's wife began the same slow process of becoming more sure of herself. The family slowly moved to a slightly higher level of differentiation. The family is a different organism when a leader emerges spontaneously from within the family. (p. 369)

This brief example captures the process which occurs when one member begins to function "more out of self" and less in reaction to the other members. When one can "rise up" out of the family oneness, the family begins to function at a better level. Significant stress will trigger an automatic pull toward togetherness in the family. This can be adaptive in the short term, but over time can result in an increased stuck togetherness, constricting the functioning of the system and its members. When a family goes through a period of regression, it is an individual who initiates a move toward better functioning and not the family unit. Family relationship patterns are fairly predictable and even more predictable when the family togetherness and resulting emotional reactivity increase. Variability in the adaptive capacity of individuals and families and how effectively they function can be most clearly observed during periods of heightened stress. This capacity, again, becomes established over the course of development for individuals and for families over the course of multiple generations.

Just as the human brain is not a tabula rasa at birth, each generation exists as part of a multigenerational process shaping the adaptive capacity of families in the present. And just as individuals do not function as autonomous beings, the adaptive capacity of families is influenced by the degree to which they are connected to the broader extended family. Isolated nuclear families are more vulnerable to the development of symptoms (Bowen, 1978; Klever, 2015). The concepts of the multigenerational emotional process and emotional cutoff will be the subjects of the next two chapters. Homo sapiens is a remarkably adaptive species. Struggle is inherent to life and the evolution of the brain and family are central to our adaptiveness as a species and in our day-to-day lives.

The residents of Bwa Mawego experienced physical and emotional stress both during hurricane Maria and in the weeks and months to follow. Their response to this event is a testament to their adaptive capacity as a community. Two years later, it was evident that there were individual differences in how well individuals and families adapted. Some adults and children continue to have heightened fear responses when non-threatening storms pass over the village, while others appear to have less reactive responses. It seems clear that the family connectedness played a key role in the recovery of individuals. If Bowen theory is accurate, variation in adaptiveness would be related to their current and multigenerational family emotional processes.

Chapter 7

Family and the Multigenerational Process

The observation that the human family functioned as a highly interdependent system shaping the development of offspring, along with the observation that the maturation of offspring varied based on their position in the family and family dynamics, led to another observation by Bowen. Variation in the adaptive capacity of families and individuals was found to be a product of multiple generations. In expanding the observational lens from the family unit to include the families of the parents and preceding generations, a novel discovery was made by Bowen. In a sense, individual development can be thought of as not beginning at conception but as conception occurring in a multigenerational context. Variation in the maturational process is shaped in the nuclear family unit, but each unit itself is shaped by the preceding generations in a predictable pattern. The multigenerational family process, as defined in Bowen theory, is posited as existing in all socioeconomic groups, in all cultures, and across the millennia. The multigenerational process is seen as influenced by the larger environment in which it unfolds but is posited to occur in all environments. The level of maturity attained by individuals over the course of development is defined in the concept of differentiation of self (Bowen, 1978). The differentiation of a self is related to the parents' level of differentiation, which in turn is found to be related to their parents' levels and so on through the generations. Once this phenomenon could be observed in families, the multigenerational family process was seen as central to the range of adaptive capacity of individuals found in the broader population. If accurate, the concept added a new dimension in the understanding of development and human behavior. Individual development, from the perspective of Bowen theory, is a multigenerational phenomenon with each generation being foundational to the next (Noone, 2014).

A simple way of describing the process is that after conception the embryo and its development is completely dependent on the maternal uterine environment. Following birth, increasing levels of independence occur over the course of development. This unfolding process is shaped by genetic, epigenetic, and environmental interactions; the family relationship system being the principal developmental environment. In the context of the interactional processes occurring in the family, the level of physical and emotional dependence on the principal caretakers declines as the child assumes more responsibility and an increasing capacity to self-regulate and move out into the broader world. On reaching adulthood, emotional autonomy or differentiation of self may vary among siblings but it is never complete. Some level of what Bowen described as unresolved emotional attachment to the caretakers remains throughout life for all in varying degrees. A consistent observation, though not yet proven, is that the degree of unresolved emotional attachment is involved in mate selection as individuals seek to bond with someone at a similar level of emotional autonomy or maturity. The level of unresolved emotional dependence of the new mating pair establishes the level of "oneness" in the formation of a new family unit in the next generation. The family oneness is shaped by the level of emotional dependence the marital pair has on one another, which in turn establishes the baseline of interdependence for the new family unit. This process proceeds over the generations. Environmental conditions, cultural norms, and life events may influence the process. Immigration, for example, may delay the age at which individuals will mate as well as influence when they will have children and how many. It may also contribute to an increase in the next generation's isolation from the extended family and so influence the pace and intensity of the multigenerational process.

A significant step in the effort to reduce subjectivity in the study of human behavior occurred when Bowen shifted the focus of the NIMH Family Study Project from the mother–child dyad to the family unit (Bowen, 2013a; Rakow, in press). This expansion of the observational lens led to the discovery of the father's participation and influence in the interactional process between mother and child. The initial hypothesis of the study was that schizophrenia developed in the intense mother–child symbiosis (Bowen, 2013a). Mother's immaturity and emotional dependency were believed to result in a failure of the dyad to emotionally separate, thus constraining the child's development. The observation, during the study, of father's part in contributing to and being an integral part of the family "oneness" allowed Bowen to see a different level of relationship process occurring—the functioning of an integrated unit. The parents were assessed to have similar levels of maturity and in degree, only slightly more than that of their child with schizophrenia. Each member could now be seen as participating in an orderly interactive process. This broader lens allowed for a significantly different understanding of the role each played in maintaining stable patterns in the relationship system. The shift from the dyad to the triangle led to a new level of systems thinking.

The inclusion of siblings living on the research unit also led to a number of new observations and research questions. How, for example, was it possible for the siblings of the schizophrenic to have attained higher levels of maturity while growing up in the same family? Now that they also lived on the research unit, it was possible to observe that the siblings were less involved in the oneness or fusion of their families (Bowen, 2013a). The observation of differences in the levels of maturity among siblings as well as Bowen's observation of variation in the levels of maturity among the research staff eventually contributed to the development of the concepts of differentiation of self and triangles. It also led to questions regarding parents' own development in their own families of origin. During the NIMH study, Bowen began to think about schizophrenia as involving more than the immediate family unit following a remark in 1955 by one of the study's consultants, Lewis Hill, that it may require three generations for schizophrenia to develop (Bowen, 1978 p. 69n).

One aspect of human subjectivity has been the tendency to see ourselves and our experiential world as central. The scientific effort has resulted in the erosion of this tendency. Our planet is no longer viewed as the center of the universe. Our sun has been found to be one of the countless stars and our species one of many to have evolved over several billion years. While the human has gained some objectivity about our place in the vast cosmos, the gains have been slower with regards to understanding our own behavior.

A hallmark of optimal maturity for an individual is the growing awareness that he or she is not the center of one's relationship world; that others are distinct selves with their own separate experiences. At the same time maturity entails a recognition of our dependence on others and the influence they have on our thoughts, feelings, and behavior as well as the influence we have on them. The observation that we function interdependently in our family emotional system, to the degree posited in Bowen theory, is still not largely recognized. It is not an easy one to grasp or accept given the individualistic perspective in the culture.

The study of the multigenerational family by Bowen led to the observation that not only do we function interdependently in our immediate families and in our families of origin, but that we and our families are products of a multigenerational past. A view that we are connected to the previous generations has existed over the millennia, with many cultures venerating their ancestral heritage. But Bowen discovered the emotional patterns operating in the multigenerational family, repeating in each generation with some variation and greatly shaping how we and our families function. The study of families with schizophrenia, of families functioning at higher levels, and of the multigenerational histories of a small number of families resulted in the observation that each family in each generation appeared to generate individual differences in the degree to which their children move toward maturity or emotional autonomy. The refinement of the concepts of differentiation of self and the nuclear family projection process shed light on how this variation occurred and the myriad ways in which it is manifested.

Following the research study, between 1959 and 1962, Bowen began a detailed multigenerational research study of a few families, with one going back more than 300 years. It was during this period that Bowen decided to do a multigenerational study of his own family. He wrote,

> Until that time I knew no more about my family than most people do of theirs: fair knowledge about grandparents, and sparse knowledge about great-grandparents. In six generations one is the product of 64 families of origin. . . . Since the early 1960s I have developed reasonable knowledge about 20 of my 64 families of origin for periods that range from 100 to 300 years. (Bowen, 1978 p. xv)

The development of the concept of differentiation of self provided a way to assess variation among individuals in the degree of maturity they attained over a life course. Based on the gathering of factual information, a consistent observation was that siblings have some variation in their basic levels of differentiation. In families with multiple siblings, some will have levels similar to that of their parents. One may reach adulthood with a level of maturity slightly higher than the parents, while most families will have at least one child who develops less maturity or adaptive capacity than his or her siblings.

The concept of the family projection process describes a family pattern in which the development of one child is more constricted than the others. The process can be expressed in a variety of ways, but at a basic level it entails the overinvolvement of a child in the parental relationship. As mentioned earlier, this emotional pattern can have a stabilizing effect for the mother, father, and the unit, but it results in the child emerging from the unit with less adaptive capacity than the other siblings. Bowen believed that the pattern was sufficiently important that it was defined as a separate concept. In describing the family projection process, he wrote,

> This is the process by which parents project part of their immaturity to one or more children. The most frequent pattern is one which operates through the mother with the mechanism which enables the mother to become less anxious by focusing on the child. The lifestyle of parents, fortuitous circumstances such as traumatic events that disrupt the family during the pregnancy or about the time of birth, and special relationships with sons or daughters are among factors

that help determine the "selection" of the child for this process. The most common pattern is one in which one child is the recipient of a major portion of the projection, while other children are relatively less involved. The child who is the object of the projection is the one most emotionally attached to the parents, and the one who ends up with a lower level of differentiation of self. A child who grows up relatively outside of the family projection process can emerge with a higher basic level of differentiation than the parents. (Bowen, 1978 p. 477)

I have not seen a family in which the projection process is not evident except perhaps in some families with an only child and in which the other adaptive mechanisms are predominant. In such families the only child may reach adulthood with a level of differentiation similar to the parents. In some families, the projection process is the principal adaptive pattern, while in others marital distance, conflict, or impairment of a spouse may be predominant. Most families have some mix of all of them. The maturational development of a child is most constricted when the projection process is the primary adaptive mechanism used by a family.

A number of variables are involved in determining which child becomes the focus of this process. In some families, generational patterns exist which may include the birth order and/or the sex of a child. For example, the oldest child might in some families be the most vulnerable and in some either a male or female child might become the focus. An oldest son may become the object of the projection process in a pattern that has continued over generations even though he may be a middle child with older sisters. Another factor in the selection of one child in the projection process may be the level of stress a family is experiencing before and after the birth of a child, resulting in the parents focusing their anxiety on that child. Other contributing factors can be seen with the careful multigenerational history of a family. In those families in which the family undifferentiation is greatest or in those experiencing prolonged and intense stress, an additional sibling may also become a focus, resulting in that child also emerging with a lower level of differentiation than the parents.

It is relatively easy to trace a decline in the adaptive capacity of families by tracking the least adaptive child in each family over several generations. The least mature child will marry at a similar level of maturity and they will produce a child with less maturity than themselves. In some generations, this process will be less pronounced than in others, but it is a predictable process found in all families. Over a number of generations, this process will predictably result in the severe impairment and loss of adaptive capacity of one or more members. Anyone can test this concept by doing a detailed multigenerational history of their own family. It can be difficult in some families to attain detailed data over more than four generations, but the process can even be observed in some families over a span of just three generations.

When a family history with sufficient data is tracked over multiple generations, most offspring can be observed to emerge with levels of adaptive capacity similar to the parents while some may be found to emerge with higher levels. But most families will produce a child with less adaptive capacity than the parents. Again, in Bowen theory, adaptive capacity is defined in the concept of differentiation of self. An individual's level of differentiation is assessed based on their functioning in a range of areas in his or her life. One child may grow up to be significantly more successful than the parents or siblings with regards to their financial status or professional accomplishments, for example. They may, however, have a severely dysfunctional spouse or child who expresses the family's undifferentiation. In observing the reciprocal functioning of family members, one member may function at a higher level in some areas, but their functioning is based on the under-functioning of another.

A measure of an individual's level of differentiation involves the functioning of their family unit as well as themselves. An example would be a family in which the emotional dependence in the marriage may be managed by a father who responds to the marital fusion with distance and primary involvement in his work life. The mother may manage the fusion with an anxious overinvolvement with a child. Each member contributes to the family emotional process. A father's distance, for example, may follow a birth and mother's involvement with that child perceiving the involvement as a decrease in her emotional involvement with him. A mother's involvement with her child can, in turn, then be influenced by the husband's distancing. The functioning of each individual in this triangle is reciprocally influenced by the functioning of the others. As mentioned, this process can have a stabilizing influence for the nuclear family but results in one child absorbing more of the family's undifferentiation. In this case, barring events which contribute to a parental projection onto another child, it is predictable that the child in this central triangle will emerge from the family with a lower level of adaptive capacity than the other siblings. The other siblings benefit due to being less constrained by the family oneness over the course of their development, allowing for a level of maturity greater than the sibling most involved in the parental triangle. One of the more fascinating discoveries made by Bowen is that, the multigenerational family process generates a wide range of adaptive capacity among the descendants of each family. As a universal process the multigenerational family process is viewed as accounting for the wide range of functioning found in the larger population.

Bowen's theory of the family emotional system and the concept of the multigenerational transmission process represented another shift away from an individual's subjective view of self and that individual's adaptive capacity. Individuals can be seen to represent not only almost four billion years of genetic transmission and natural selection but as occupying a functional position in a multigenerational family process. The development of the concept of the multigenerational family transmission process describes a relationship process generating the differential development of siblings occurring in each family unit over multiple generations. His observation was that this multigenerational process entailed more than genes:

> My concept, multigenerational transmission process, defines a very broad pattern in which certain children emerge with lower levels of differentiation than the parents, and others emerge with higher levels of differentiation, while most continue at about the same level as the parents. . . . From a strict definition of genetics, this process follows a genetic-like pattern but it has nothing to do with genes as they are currently defined. (Bowen, 1978 pp. 410–411)

Since the time Bowen developed the concept of the multigenerational transmission process more than 60 years ago, a revolution in the understanding of genetics and their expression has occurred. At the time, the predominant view was that even though the environment or "nurture" influenced phenotypic development, genes or "nature" functioned somewhat independently and in a unidirectional manner. In recent decades, however, the rapidly developing field of epigenetics has transformed the knowledge of gene–environment interactions. The nature/nurture dichotomy is no longer so dichotomous (Meaney, 2010). The discovery of epigenetic processes has provided evidence for how the family emotional system can have such a profound effect on the physiology, behavior, and lifetime functioning of individuals.

EPIGENETICS AND MULTIGENERATIONAL FAMILY TRANSMISSION

During several decades following Bowen's family research, many in psychiatry and the neurosciences believed schizophrenia was "biological," a neurological disorder largely developed independently of the family. Much attention was focused on the search for the genetic cause of the disease and its pharmaceutical treatment (Bentall, 2004). A common misunderstanding was that if a phenomenon like schizophrenia was biological it must be genetic. In a relatively brief period, psychiatry abandoned the idea that the family or social environment might play a role in the development of schizophrenia. This view was extended to other diagnoses such as depression, bipolar, and other disorders.

The "central dogma" in biology held that genetic information encoded in DNA contained the blueprint for the developing phenotype. DNA was transcribed to messenger RNA which then translated the information to produce proteins, the building blocks of the phenotype. With the exception of reverse transcription, in which RNA could provide some feedback to the DNA, it was seen as a one-way process. DNA was believed to be uninfluenced by proteins or the individual phenotype.

For decades, the expression, nature versus nurture, was used to describe the genetic and environmental influences on child development. They were thought to be separate factors shaping individual differences. Genes were believed to be the units of inheritance and a basic assumption in this view was that no other biological factors were involved in heredity. It has since become apparent, however, that the genome cannot function independently of its environmental context (Boyce & Kobor, 2015; Meaney, 2010). Based on both animal and human studies, knowledge developing in the field of epigenetics has greatly expanded the view of what is involved in familial transmission.

In what might have been thought of as heretical only a few decades ago, is now evident as Michael Meaney, a prominent investigator in the field of epigenetics, writes:

> While there are indeed statistical relations between variation in nucleotide sequence and that in complex traits, at the level of biology there are no genes for intelligence, depression, athletic abilities, fashion sense, or any other such complex trait. . . . There are multiple and complex cellular processes that lie between the DNA sequence and the functional outcome associated with the gene product. (Meaney, 2010, p. 45)

The genome of an individual organism is now known to interact with both the cellular and larger environment and its functioning is modifiable based on those contexts. The epigenetic regulation of DNA does not alter the sequence of the information it contains, but it does play an important role in determining which genes are expressed or silenced. An individual's experiences, especially during sensitive periods of development such as intrauterine, neonatal, and adolescence, can result in biochemical signaling which can modify gene expression (Champagne, 2011; Crews & Noone, 2015; Szyf et al., 2008). In recent decades, animal and human studies have provided evidence that the parent–offspring relationship can epigenetically influence brain development and behavior of offspring and that this influence can extend over several generations (Curley & Champagne, 2016). The emerging field of epigenetics has transformed knowledge of biological inheritance and contributed to an understanding of how the multigenerational family emotional process could have such a profound effect (Jones, 2014; Lassiter, 2020). As researchers Michael Meaney and Moshe Szyf (2005) write in discussing the impact of epigenetic changes induced by parental care: "Indeed, maternal effects could result in the transmission of adaptive responses across generations. In humans, such effects might contribute to the familial transmission of risk and resilience" (p. 462).

Two of the more studied epigenetic processes relevant to the concept of the multigenerational transmission process described in Bowen theory are those involved in shaping stress reactivity and parental care. A series of elegant studies by Michael Meaney and his colleagues at McGill University (Francis et al., 1999; Champagne, 2008; Zhang & Meaney, 2010) provided evidence that variation in maternal care among rats induced epigenetic lifelong changes in the stress reactivity of offspring. Cross-fostering offspring further provided the evidence that it was the maternal care and not the mother's biology that resulted in the changes. The offspring of mothers highly reactive to stress when placed with low-reactive mothers became low-reactive adults. Similarly, the offspring of low-reactive mothers became high reactors as adults if they had been placed and reared with high-reactive mothers. The changes in the hypothalamic–pituitary–adrenal (HPA) neuroendocrine stress response system were found to be transmitted not only from mother to offspring but over multiple generations. The offspring of cross-fostered pups inherited the same epigenetic changes as their mothers.

The epigenetic transmission of changes in the HPA stress response system involves the density of receptors for the stress hormone glucocorticoid (GR) in the hippocampus. The hippocampus plays a vital role in the regulation of the HPA stress response system. As mentioned previously, the HPA system, in response to a perceived threat, releases glucocorticoids (cortisol in humans) into the bloodstream, upregulating and downregulating the physiological systems involved in effectively responding to challenge. When picked up by receptors in the hippocampus, it signals the HPA system to cease producing the stress hormone. As the prolonged elevation of cortisol can lead to a less effective stress response system and the development of stress-related symptoms, this regulatory function serves as an important factor in health and well-being.

Variation in parental care was found to be related to whether the genes for GR were expressed or silenced (Weaver et al., 2004). The greater the density of GR in the hippocampus, the more effective the regulation of the HPA system. The genes for GR in the high-reactive mothers were found to be silenced by a process called "methylation." This results in a less effective regulation of the HPA system and a prolonged elevation of stress hormones (Meaney, 2010). The cross-fostering of pups at birth showed that this process was not genetically but epigenetically transferred from mother to offspring. In terms of the multigenerational transmission of adaptive capacity of individuals, this research has provided some support for how the functioning of the family emotional system can influence the physiological, emotional, and behavioral functioning of offspring from generation to generation (Jones, 2014; Lassiter, 2020; Noone, 2015).

In addition to variation in maternal care contributing to the epigenetic transmission of stress reactivity of offspring, the epigenetic transmission of parental care itself has also been found (Champagne, 2011; Curley & Champagne, 2016). The experimental stressing of rodent mothers has been found to influence the maternal care of their daughters. At the molecular level, maternal care not only results in the expression or silencing of genes regulating stress reactivity in offspring but in genes involved in parental care. As Champagne (2011) writes,

> Interestingly, one of the consequences of variation in the experience of maternal care is in the development of neuroendocrine circuits which will shape the subsequent maternal and reproductive behavior of female offspring. Through this process, a transmission of individual differences in maternal behavior can be achieved. (p. 4)

Maternal care has been found to result in the expression or silencing of the genes for hypothalamic estrogen receptors in female offspring. The females receiving low levels of maternal care and thus fewer estrogen receptors provide less maternal care to their offspring and this behavior was found to persist over multiple generations (Champagne & Curley, 2015).

While much remains unknown about the epigenetic transmission of behavioral traits related to the adaptive capacity of offspring, it is clear that environmental and especially familial factors interact with the genomes of individuals and the effects of such factors can influence adaptive capacity over multiple generations. The multigenerational transmission process as defined in Bowen theory involves more than the epigenetic processes affecting the expression of genes influencing the physiology and behavior of offspring. But the evidence from the animal and human study of epigenetic transmission provides support for how parental care can have such a profound effect at the biological level and how that effect can be transmitted over the generations.

In describing the dramatic change which has occurred in the understanding of nature–nurture interactions based on epigenetic studies Champagne (2011) writes,

> An emerging theme in these studies is the significant change in gene expression within the brain which can arise in response to environmental experiences occurring during the early stages of development. Evidence for

environmentally-induced changes in transcriptional activity has triggered an evolution in our understanding of the interplay between genes and the environment. Rather than being constrained by the nature-nurture debate, we are rapidly moving forward and developing hypotheses that consider the common biological pathways through which genes and the environment operate. (p. 5)

In addition to the epigenetic effects being transmitted from generation to generation, the influence of the relationship environment on genetic expression has also been discovered to exist throughout an individual's lifespan. A field of study described as social genomics is providing evidence that a portion of our genomes are sensitive to social interactions which can result in their being expressed or silenced. As investigators George Slavich and Steven Cole at UCLA write,

This research on human social genomics has begun to identify the types of genes that are subject to social-environmental regulation, the neural and molecular mechanisms that mediate the effects of social processes on gene expression, and the genetic polymorphisms that moderate individual differences in genomic sensitivity to social context. The molecular models resulting from this research provide new opportunities for understanding how social and genetic factors interact to shape complex behavioral phenotypes and susceptibility to disease. This research also sheds new light on the evolution of the human genome and challenges the fundamental belief that our molecular makeup is relatively stable and impermeable to social-environmental influence. (Slavich & Cole, 2013)

The lifelong epigenetic processes appear to be particularly influenced as a result of the impact of parental care on offspring brain development. As Curley and Champagne (2016) write,

Though it had been assumed that epigenetic alterations had limited plasticity beyond the early stages of embryonic development, there is increasing evidence that these processes are highly dynamic throughout the lifespan in response to a variety of environmental signals. In particular, variation in the quality and/or quantity of maternal care is associated with epigenetic variation in the brain of offspring. (p. 58)

In summary, the concept of the multigenerational family process describes the family's influence in shaping the development of a self among offspring in each generation. The differentiation of a self as defined in Bowen theory involves genetic, epigenetic, physiological, psychological, and relationship variables which shape the degree of maturation individuals attain over the course of development. Each generation generates some variation in the maturational process and the variation is carried forward into the next generation. Just as the brain at birth is not a blank slate, each family does not begin anew. Each family must adapt to its environment and its capacity to adapt rests to a significant degree on the adaptiveness of the preceding generation. Though the environment as well as life's good fortunes or misfortunes are influential, the differentiation of a self appears to be a relatively stable process. The concept of the family multigenerational process has not yet been adequately tested, but knowledge developing in the sciences, along with the multigenerational research by a significant number of individuals with their own families, provides evidence for its continued study. If accurate, the shaping of variation in the adaptive capacity of families and individuals by the multigenerational family process will represent a significant advance in the understanding of human behavior.

Chapter 8

Emotional Cutoff and the Establishment of a Self in Each Generation

The concept of differentiation of self in Bowen theory captures the central evolutionary development contributing to the remarkable adaptive capacity found in Homo sapiens. The evolution of the complex human brain increased the individual's capacity to self-regulate and to be self-directed. The dramatic expansion of the neocortex and especially the prefrontal cortex in the hominin line involved an increased capacity to regulate the more automatic emotional system allowing for greater flexibility in responding to the social and physical environments. In addition to enabling our species to create and live in larger and more complex social systems (Dunbar, 2016), this evolutionary development has permitted the human to respond more effectively to the social environment, allowing for such abilities as theory of mind, social competence, shared intentionality, and hyper-cooperativity (Burkart, Hrdy, & van Shaik, 2009; Flinn, Quinlan, Coe, & Ward, 2007). The increase in the complexity of the prefrontal cortex, according to Fuster (2013), permitted Homo sapiens to not only adapt to present environmental challenges but to "pre-adapt" by visualizing potential scenarios to be responded to. The concept of differentiation of self is a developmental concept which describes the variation in levels of maturity attained by individuals, which, according to Bowen theory, involves the maturation of the higher cortical systems. It is posited that the maturation or differentiation of the higher cortical systems permits a greater capacity to more objectively appraise the relationship environment.

As mentioned in chapter 4, the evolution of our complex brains went hand-in-glove with the evolution of the highly integrated unit of the family. The enhanced ability to self-regulate also involved the evolution of the higher-level, self-regulating system of the family. It is in this context that the differentiation of self develops during the first two decades of life. The human family provides the protective environment necessary for a prolonged period of brain development and a complex relationship system in which a developing child can learn the social skills required to navigate in the larger social environment. It is also the environment in which individuals mature and attain varying degrees of an emotionally autonomous self.

The lengthy period of brain growth, particularly, that of the cerebral cortex, greatly enhanced the capacity for learning about the present environment, distinguishing between it and previous experiences of the environment. The family provided the necessary context for the acquisition of the amazing linguistic skills found in Homo sapiens along with an increased capacity to transmit knowledge from one generation to the next. In the midst of the heightened interdependence and co-regulation involved in the integrated family system, the development of the higher cortical systems created the potential for a greater capacity to manage oneself. And finally, the highly integrated family system and complex brain increased greater responsiveness to social signals, social tolerance, and cooperative behavior, characteristics vital to the growth of larger social systems.

In addition to describing variation in the development of the intellectual system, the concept of differentiation of self also entails the related developmental process of emotionally separating from the family of origin and establishing an adult life course. The development of the intellectual system and the differentiation of a separate self are related and central to the adaptive capacity of individuals. Likewise, the degree to which an individual remains emotionally dependent on the family of origin determines the degree to which the relationship system regulates his or her behavior. An individual's level of emotional dependence determines how predominant the more automatic emotional system is or how much choice or flexibility one has in responding to environmental challenges. It is this intermix between the emotional and intellectual systems that occurs over the course of development that establishes an individual's level of differentiation (Noone, 2016).

From both an evolutionary and developmental perspective, the ideal or even adequate construction of the complex brain found in Homo sapiens requires membership in the prolonged, protective, and interactive system of the family. As previously mentioned, the evolution of the family is viewed not simply as a result of cultural evolution but as a biological development entailing the biological substrates selected for in maintaining the intricate and long-lasting bonds found in the human family (Fleming, 2005; Flinn, Ward, & Noone, 2005).

The developing human brain evolved to require the active engagement of parental caretakers and other members of the immediate and extended family (Allman, 1999). At the same time there is a cost involved in this membership, a cost associated with emotional dependence. Murray Bowen's study of the family led to the observation that family members are more deeply attached to one another than most are willing to admit. The construction of a self begins in the warmth of the uterine environment, where for nine months the assemblage and differentiation of cells result in the birth of an altricial infant. But during its intrauterine development, the embryo is not isolated from the larger environment. Even before the embryo begins to hear sounds, mother's interactions in the social arena can be communicated through neuroendocrine signaling. At birth, though still dependent, the infant begins the lengthy process of attaining increasing levels of autonomy, starting with the ability to breathe and thermoregulate on its own. Development continues, but from the very beginning it involves the family emotional system. Jennifer Barrett and Alison Fleming (2011) capture some of this interactive process in writing:

> Romanticism aside, the mother-offspring dance is influenced by and interacts with many factors, including mothers' physiology, cultural and family context, maternal cognitions, maternal affect and stress and the early environment, notably a mother's own early experiences in her family of origin. Biological influences certainly include how mothers' brains are organized and how genes and environment interact in brain development. (p. 368)

Bowen theory, of course, holds that the mother–offspring dance is part of the larger dance occurring in the family. The family dance of reciprocal influencing reflects the underlying interdependence at play as each member's functioning contributes to the functioning of each other and the larger whole. Over the course of development, the level of emotional maturity attained by individuals is largely regulated by an unfolding dance shaped by the current and multigenerational family process as well as the environmental reality to which the family is adapting.

Offspring mature to varying degrees, but no individual attains complete emotional autonomy. Family oneness varies among families, but all families can be found to maintain a level of oneness or emotional interdependence beyond the developmental years of offspring. On reaching adulthood, individuals are faced with the task of moving out into the world and pursuing their own course in life. In doing so, each person must manage their own emotional dependence on their families as they separate. From the perspective of Bowen theory, the remaining dependence or undifferentiation each individual has on reaching adulthood will influence their functioning and adaptive capacity throughout their adult life.

The process of growing into young adulthood and assuming responsibility for one's life is a fascinating phenomenon. It is a process influencing adaptive capacity and includes mate selection and the establishment of a family in the next generation. It is also a process determining the quality and extent of the ongoing relationships between the generations, the extent to which they can remain in viable contact over the years. Central to the extent to which young adults and their parents separate is the degree of what Bowen described as the level of unresolved emotional attachment remaining in their relationships. In meeting the demands of adult life, each generation must grapple with the struggle between the biological and psychological drives to become independent and the degree to which they remain embedded in the family oneness which continues to exist. As Bowen (1978) writes,

> One of the most important functional patterns in a family has to do with the intensity of the unresolved emotional attachment to parents, most frequently to the mother for both men and women, and the way the individual handles the attachment. . . . However the issue is handled, the denied emotional attachment to the past replicates itself with one's spouse and one's children. This can be said another way: The more one denies the attachment to the past, the less choice one has in determining the pattern with his own wife and children (as if he has much choice to begin with). (p. 433)

As Bowen described it, one aspect of how this emotional dependence is managed involves a degree of denial of the unresolved attachment, accompanied by a feeling of being more adult or independent than one's functioning indicates. Given this denial and the many forms and environmental contexts in which the separation between the generations occurs, it is difficult to assess the level of unresolved emotional dependence of individuals without knowledge of the concept of differentiation of self. In pretending to be more independent than one is, individuals can appear to be more emotionally separate than is the case. A careful assessment of an individual's level of differentiation of self, which includes many variables, provides a more accurate view than would be captured by an individual's self-report.

The level of an individual's unresolved emotional attachment is largely equivalent to his or her level of differentiation of self. It is also influenced by how parents have managed higher levels of anxiety occurring during important times in development of their children. Bowen described the influence differentiation of self and anxiety have in shaping the level of unresolved emotional attachment of individuals in writing:

> The degree of unresolved emotional attachment to parents is determined by the degree of unresolved emotional attachment each parent had in their own family of origin, the way their parents handled this in their marriage, the degree of anxiety during critical periods in life, and the way the parents handled this anxiety. . . . There is a variable determined by the ways parents handle anxiety. In broad terms, the amount of anxiety tends to parallel the degree of unresolved emotional attachment in the family. For instance, a family with a higher level

of undifferentiation will be a more disorganized family with higher levels of anxiety, and a family with better levels of differentiation will be more orderly with lower levels of anxiety. Families in which the parents handle anxiety well, and in which they are able to stay on a predetermined course in spite of anxiety, will turn out better than the families in which the parents are more reactive and shift life courses in response to anxiety. All things being equal, the life course of people is determined by the amount of unresolved emotional attachment, the amount of anxiety that comes from it, and the way they deal with this anxiety. (Bowen, 1978 pp. 536–537)

Murray Bowen developed the concept of emotional cutoff to describe the emotional process between generations and the manner in which the unresolved attachment to the past is handled. The concept describes the emotional distancing an individual requires to function as an adult. The distance represents a way of decreasing the emotional sensitivity parents and an adult child experience due to their remaining emotional dependence as they interact. The emotional sensitivity parents and their children experience with each other can be observed throughout development. From infancy through adolescence, parents and child are continuously responding to one another as they react to the pressures resulting from the demands of dependency and the effort to gain autonomy. An infant will cry to be picked up and comforted as well as wiggle to be released and be separate. A mother may react with frustration to the demands of an infant or seek the comfort she can experience in intimately bonding with her child. An adolescent may feel constrained by the family oneness and react with distance or conflict. He may also seek to be engaged and connect in numerous ways. A parent may react to his son's distancing or distance himself when the relationship becomes more intense.

It can be difficult to comprehend the function of emotional cutoff without an appreciation of the depth of attachment processes which exist in the family throughout the life cycle. The observation that the family functions as a unit and that the interdependence of its members entails biological substrates as well as psychological and relationship processes provide some understanding of the depth of family connectedness and the adaptive function entailed in emotionally cutting off. On reaching adulthood, offspring and parental caretakers must necessarily separate in order to move into the future and establish a new generation. Since family units vary in the degree of emotional oneness, so too will the level of emotional cutoff required in order to separate.

Adolescence is often a period when the interplay between an offspring's emerging autonomy and remaining emotional dependence is most observable. Biological and emotional processes characteristically are involved in an adolescent's effort to lift off. Based on the level of emotional dependence or undifferentiation between parents and their child, this can be a relatively smooth process or one of emotional turbulence. At greater levels of maturity, parents and their adolescent are less reactive to the development of more autonomy. The adolescent is more responsible and less anxious about moving into the broader social world. The parents are more realistic about the moves for more independence and the relationships remain more open and mutually respectful. Their capacity for managing the anxieties involved in the process of separating is based more on the reality of the son's or daughter's current level of development than projected fears about the dangers involved in gaining autonomy.

At lower levels of maturity, adolescence can be a period of heightened reactivity. The adolescent imperative to be more independent can be experienced as a threat. Parents may have more difficulty in separating from their son or daughter, not recognizing their own dependence on their child. The adolescent may also be less confident in assuming more responsibility, struggling between the push and pulls of autonomy and dependence. This can result in an escalation of over-parental behavior in response to some of their child's immature behavior, and the adolescent's emotionally reacting to parental constraints with an increase in defiant or less responsible behavior. Parents may unconsciously experience the family oneness as being threatened, while the adolescent may feel both their autonomy and dependence to be threatened. The increased level of emotional reactivity then results in a less open parent–child relationship expressed with increased distance and/or conflict.

One family described their concern about their son's recent increased irresponsibility. He was in his last semester senior year in high school. They stated he had always been highly responsible and successful academically and socially. Now they found him to be acting less maturely. As son became less responsible, father had become more "parental." And as father became more parental, son became more infantile. In discussing their concerns, the parents began to wonder whether they might all be becoming more anxious about the son's departure for college in the fall. Once they could begin to see their own anxiety about this anticipated separation, they could see with some humor their own reactivity. As they relaxed a bit and became less parental, their son began to return to his more mature self.

Greater levels of emotional dependence can also result in the opposite scenario. Rather than rebel, an adolescent might respond to the family tension created by the pressures entailed in separating from the family oneness by remaining in a more compliant childlike state. This results in less conflict or overt reactivity between the parents and their child but creates more difficulties in later adolescence when a separation may be required, such as leaving for college or joining the military. At an extreme, it can take the form of a functional collapse and a return to the family home, or the development of depression or a substance abuse problem.

From the perspective of Bowen theory, development involves a process of an offspring attaining increasing levels of a self in the context of the relationship environment, of which the caretakers are central. The differentiation of a self entails the movement toward an increasing capacity to self-regulate and be self-directed in the relationship system. It involves the relative capacity to think for oneself even when the family or group exerts some pressure to think alike. A universal dilemma faced by individuals as they move into adulthood is the challenge of managing the remaining unresolved emotional dependency, and the concept of emotional cutoff describes the universal process of the attempt to do so.

Some degree of emotional cutoff can be observed in each generation. Knowledge of Bowen theory and a detailed multigenerational study of the family provides evidence of the varying degrees of maturity attained by offspring in each generation. The principal factors contributing to the level of maturity individuals attain influence the process of emotionally separating from the family as an adult. This includes the parents' level of maturity, the family's emotional patterns, and environmental factors. This process and its influence on the adaptive capacity of individuals can be observed over the generations as each generation is influenced by the degree to which the previous generation managed to emotionally separate from their family of origin. The degree to which parents have cut off from their families will influence the process of their own children's separation and so it is accurate to say that the degree of emotional cutoff among family members has been generations in the making (Bowen, 2017). In a very real sense, we inherit some degree of emotional cutoff from the previous generations.

The higher the level of differentiation or maturity an individual has attained, the less emotional cutoff he or she will have with the parents. The development of a more solid self allows a person to be in viable contact with his or her parents. Their relationship will remain more open and involve less emotional reactivity related to differences they might have. At greater levels of maturity, individuals have more choice in the amount and quality of contact they have with each other. They may be geographically distant or live nearby, but they remain in good contact during both calm and challenging times.

Though emotional cutoff is roughly equivalent to an individual's level of unresolved emotional attachment or differentiation, some differences among individuals at similar levels can be observed in how the unresolved attachment is handled. Bowen (1978) described the impact some of these differences can have on the adaptive capacity of families:

> The more a nuclear family maintains some kind of viable emotional contact with the past generations, the more orderly and asymptomatic the life process in both

generations. Compare two families with identical levels of differentiation. One family remains in contact with the parental family and remains relatively free of symptoms for life, and the level of differentiation does not change much in the next generation. The other family cuts off with the past, develops symptoms and dysfunction, and a lower level of differentiation in the succeeding generation. (p. 23)

Emotional cutoff is an adaptive response. It represents an effort on the part of individuals to regulate the tension involved in having a life of one's own while continuing to remain to some degree in the "family oneness." At the same time, one's level of emotional cutoff from the parental family significantly influences one's functioning in current and future relationships. A common example of this process is heard when a person describes their unhappiness with the parental care they experienced growing up. They may remain in contact with their parents but maintain distance by keeping it superficial or infrequent. They will say that in parenting their own children they will not repeat their parents' errors. They may, for example, report that their parents never provided sufficient emotional support for them as a child (though an exploration of their families often indicates a great deal of emotional involvement). As parents themselves they are dedicated to being supportive, showing up at all their child's activities, praising all their child's efforts, and intervening in their struggles to assure them they care and to help them avoid discomfort or disappointment. When this parental effort represents an emotional overinvolvement, it is not difficult to predict how their children will respond on reaching adolescence or early adulthood.

Bowen originally developed the concept of emotional cutoff to describe the process involved as the generations separate but the level of an individual's unresolved emotional attachment and the degree of cutoff required to function as an independent adult will be activated to some extent in all emotionally important relationships. Bowen (1978) writes,

> Basic relationship patterns developed for adapting to the parental family in childhood are used in all other relationships throughout life. The basic patterns in social and work relationships are identical to relationship patterns in the family, except in intensity. . . . This is more pronounced in people with lower levels of differentiation who have higher levels of unresolved emotional attachments to their parents. (p. 462)

The degree of emotional cutoff in response to the underlying unresolved emotional attachment is most apparent in response to the emotional fusion occurring in a marriage. Since people select a mate with a similar level of emotional maturity, the resulting fusion in the pair will approximate the fusion they each had with their parental relationships. It is accurate to say that the level of unresolved emotional dependence of an individual will surface again in the marital relationship.

If the proposition that individuals select a mate with a similar level of differentiation is accurate, each partner will necessarily have to adapt to a similar level of emotional dependence with the other. The concept of the nuclear family emotional process describes the adaptive patterns family units establish to manage their fusion. Depending on the level of fusion or undifferentiation involved, some level of chronic anxiety will need to be managed in the marital pair. Emotional distancing following the initial fusion is predictable in a marriage as each adapts to their dependence on one another. The degree to which each has emotionally cutoff from their families of origin will influence how they will manage their emotional dependence with one another and with their children.

Emotional cutoff can be thought of as an individual's effort to function as a self despite their degree of undifferentiation from their family of origin. But the concept is not an individual concept as it refers to a process occurring in the context of the family emotional system. It is a relationship concept and one that significantly influences the functioning of the family unit. As mentioned previously, families with similar levels of differentiation can differ in their adaptive capacity based on the degree to which they have been able to maintain some viable emotional contact with the larger extended family. Thus, an individual who manages his unresolved emotional attachment by emotionally cutting off from the larger extended family will influence the functioning of his family in the next generation. The emotional distance resulting from the cutoff will result in an increase in the isolation of a nuclear family and likely increase the level of emotional intensity in that family. In cutting off from the family of origin, an individual decreases the capacity for the extended family to be a resource and during stressful periods his or her immediate family will be more vulnerable to a buildup of tension or anxiety. As a result, families more isolated from the larger family are more vulnerable to the development of symptoms (Kerr, 2019; Klever, 2016; McKnight, 2020). The effort to establish a self by cutting off from the previous generation typically results in an individual's utilizing emotional distancing as an adaptive pattern in future emotionally important relationships. It will influence that individual's functioning and contribute to the potential for cutting off in the marriage and with one's children.

Families vary in their adaptive capacity and the degree of isolation from the larger extended and multigenerational family is one of the factors contributing to this capacity. In his family assessment model of the family, Papero (2018) posits that one of the five dimensions on which the adaptive capacity of a family can be assessed is that of connectedness and integration. He posits that this dimension refers to both "the frequency and breadth of contact and the quality of the contact" a family has with the intergenerational family. He writes,

> One can infer from Bowen's descriptions that well-functioning families present a high degree of connectedness and integration (a term Bowen used to describe the degree of openness in interpersonal relationships). A well-integrated family system would therefore include a significant percentage of person to person relationships for each family member. As a result of those relationships, family members are in good communication with each other about important matters, know to an important degree how each person sees the world and thinks about issues and challenges, and display a significant degree of tolerance and respect for each other's viewpoints. In contrast, a family with a high degree of cutoff among its members would reflect infrequent contact, incomplete communication with each other, and limited knowledge of one another's thinking. (Papero, 2018 p. 139)

According to Papero, families exist along a continuum in their degree of connectedness and integration. Families at higher levels of differentiation are generally less isolated from their larger extended families and the openness existing in those relationships is of a higher quality. The value of this connectedness is especially observable when families are going through particularly stressful periods. Following the death of a family member or a serious illness, extended family members come together providing support and comfort to the members of a family unit. Similarly, during positive events, such as a baptism or bar mitzvah, the celebrations are enriched for all when the larger family is engaged. Such gatherings reinforce the family ties going forward and provide memories of their connections. From a developmental perspective, the exposure to the larger extended family, with all of the differences, quirks, and conflicts involved, provides a child with a wider range of relationship experience and a broader view of what is entailed in family. Engagement with the larger family provides a spectrum of relationships along with a host of member reactions to one another which becomes part of a child's experience in learning how to navigate in the social arena.

Emotional cutoff can be observed to varying degrees among individuals in all multigenerational families. It can be quite subtle but can be found in its more exaggerated forms when a detailed multigenerational history is taken. Karl Pillemer at Cornell University and his colleagues have done extensive intergenerational studies on the quality of relationships between adult children and their parents from a sociological perspective (Gilligan, Suitor, & Pillemer, 2015). In approximately 11 percent of the 566 families in a full sample, mothers reported being estranged from at least one of their adult children. Such estrangements typically represent the more overt forms of cutoff. Less overt forms are found when adult offspring may maintain frequent contact with parents but keep the relationship at a superficial and impersonal level.

Bowen theory provides a conceptual framework for observing the emotional process in families and sheds light on the universal process of generations separating from each other and the degree of emotional cutoff entailed in doing so. Emotional cutoff can be adaptive in the process of separating and moving into adulthood, but still have an effect on the adaptive capacity of the next generation. Knowledge of cutoff in one's family can be useful to the motivated individual seeking to improve their adaptive capacity and that of their family.

In clinical practice, a consistent observation is that when a motivated family member can work to establish a more open relationship with extended family members and overcome what had been varying degrees of cutoff, the severity of a symptom in their nuclear family will subside. While making increased contact with extended family members by itself will not increase a person's basic level of differentiation, it will most often increase the adaptive capacity of that person and his or her immediate family. It has the potential to increase what Bowen described as one's functional level of differentiation as well as create the context for the effort to increase one's basic level of differentiation of self.

At present, it is not uncommon for many professionals in the field of mental health to advise clients to avoid what are viewed as "toxic" relationships in the family. They are generally the relationships which stir up significant anguish or conflict with one or more family members. Those members may exhibit some form of dysfunction or be overly intrusive. There may be a history of abuse or neglect which continues to result in some emotional pain. Avoiding contact with them will predictably decrease a person's anxiety, but it is generally a short-term benefit at the expense of a potential long-term gain for the individual and for the family. From a Bowen theory perspective, some distancing in a particularly difficult relationship may be useful as a temporary strategy, but only in the effort to gain some objectivity about the "toxic" family member. An approach based in Bowen theory would involve learning more facts about that person's history and their position in the larger extended and multigenerational family. It would involve learning more about the interlocking triangles which have played a role in that person's functioning and relationship involvement. Rather than cutting off from a particularly difficult relationship, a broader perspective can enable one to see that relationship as an opportunity to both learn more about the family and make gains in one's capacity to regulate self in a tension-provoking arena. For some people and some relationships, it may take several years to get to the point at which they can effectively manage themselves in such difficult relationships. When one is able to do this, they have made gains in their own capacity to regulate self, a capacity that will carry over into other relationships.

The concept of emotional cutoff describes a universal family relationship process. It may take different forms in different families and in different cultures, but it represents an adaptive response in the effort to manage one's unresolved emotional attachment to the parental family. Emotional cutoff is neither good nor bad, but simply a fact of human adaptation. It represents an adaptation resulting from the degree of oneness existing in the family. Family oneness is an element vital to the adaptiveness of families and the maturational development of individuals, but in its more exaggerated forms, it limits the potential adaptive capacity of families and individuals. There are both benefits and costs for being a member of the higher-level unit of the family adaptive system. The environment so necessary for the prolonged development of a child and effective adaptation in the larger social world can also constrict that development and functioning of that child.

Bowen theory posits that there is variation among offspring in the degree to which they mature. Maturation involves the development of an individual self. And the development of a self, according to Bowen theory, involves the maturation of the brain and its higher cortical systems (the intellectual system). A baseline for variation in the development of a self is established by the parental pair, whose level of maturity was developed in their families of origin. Based on this process, families vary in the degree to which their offspring mature or differentiate. Parents at higher levels of differentiation will have offspring varying slightly, over the course of development, in attaining emotional autonomy from the parental family. At lower levels, offspring will also vary in their development, but the increased "stuck togetherness" will constrict the degree of individuation to be attained. As mentioned earlier, the family's multigenerational process generates variation in the adaptive capacity of individuals and families, but all individuals must deal with some degree of unresolved attachment involved in their family oneness. Figure 8.1 illustrates a continuum of maturity or differentiation of self and characteristics involved, including emotional cutoff.

My own family and my effort to know extended family represented an example of the value of having a theory to explore the family and the concept of emotional cutoff to shed light on a basic process.

Each of my parents had individually emigrated as adolescents from large families in the impoverished environment of Ireland in the 1920s. Some of their siblings also emigrated and as a child I had some contact with a few members of the extended family. Travel was expensive and since the families in Ireland did not have telephones, the only communication among family members was by letter. I knew a bit about my grandparents, aunts, and uncles,

Maturation

other-regulated, other-directed   self-regulated, self-directed

$$\longleftarrow\hspace{8cm}\longrightarrow$$

• less capacity to regulate
  emotional reactivity

• less flexibility in behavioral
  responses to challenge

• higher levels of chronic anxiety

• an increase in degree of
  emotional cutoff

• more flexibility and choice in
  responding to life's challenges

• lower level of chronic anxiety

• a decrease in degree of
  emotional cutoff

Figure 8.1   Maturation and Emotional Cutoff. *Source:* Created by the author.

but not much. My parents would learn of their own parents' deaths by tele-grams and though they grieved, I learned little about their lives.

As I mentioned earlier, my clinical experience with families led to my curiosity about my own extended family. My aunts, uncles, and their families, as part of the Irish diaspora, lived in several countries. As a young adult, curious about my family, I visited most of them one summer and found the experience exhilarating. Every family I visited was welcoming and my view of family was greatly expanded. These visits were prior my gaining knowledge of Bowen theory. I had assumed that the minimal contact among family members in the larger extended family was simply due to socioeconomic factors.

Four years later, after my exposure to Bowen theory, I visited the same families. I gained a wealth of family information due to the theory which guided my effort and the gathering of family history from various aunts and uncles. In chapter 10, I describe some of the basic principles involved in the effort to differentiate in one's family, but that trip led to the recognition of some of the more obvious emotional cutoffs in the family. Over time, I also came to recognize the function that emotional cutoff played for various family members. It assisted people in establishing their lives in more hospitable environments but also impacted the functioning of the various nuclear families. The degree of emotional cutoff by an aunt or uncle could be observed to have influenced their life courses as well as that of their children.

The phenomenon of emotional cutoff thus represents an adaptive response, enabling individuals to function despite their lack of emotional separation from their parental families. It represents a response in managing one's own immaturity. Knowledge of emotional cutoff in one's self and in one's family, however, is invaluable to the person seeking to increase their level of maturity and adaptive capacity. As an adaptive response for individuals and families over the generations, overcoming the emotional cutoff in a family is not a simple task. Bowen (2017) writes,

> It is a complex process transmitted from the past. No single generation can reverse the process. Any single generation can take a few steps to decrease the intensity of the process, if people are motivated to work at it, and if they have some accurate information about the nature of the process and some clues about how to approach it. (Bowen, 2017 p. 57)

The "nature of the process," of course, includes an understanding of the emotional system and the degree of interdependency existing in the family emotional system. The theory provides "some clues about how to approach it." Emotional cutoff represents just one element of individual and family functioning and is interrelated to the other seven concepts which make up Bowen theory. As a whole Bowen theory represents a conceptual framework useful in exploring one's family and enhancing one's functioning.

Chapter 9

A Systems Theory of the Family

The use of the term "paradigm" has come to be used more loosely than it was in Thomas Kuhn's influential book *The Structure of Scientific Revolutions*, which was first published in 1962. Kuhn (2012) used the term to describe the communities of scientists or practitioners attracted to transformative ideas which led them away from the predominant modes of scientific understanding and inquiry of the time. He added that the new paradigm "was sufficiently open-ended to leave all sorts of problems for the redefined group of practitioners to resolve" (2012, 11). Though Kuhn principally referred to the physical sciences, his view of the normal process of science has been applied to the life and social sciences as well.

Apart from those involved in the "family movement" occurring during the third-quarter of the twentieth century, Bowen was unique among investigators in developing a formal theory of family systems. In the more than fifty years since its introduction, the theory has continued to be developed and practitioners have been trained in its application at various centers around the country and the world. As a natural systems theory of the family, it remains distinct from the predominantly individualistic paradigms existing in the disciplines related to human behavior. The development of knowledge in the sciences has continued, knowledge which the various disciplines and paradigms attempt in varying degrees to integrate.

While psychoanalysis may have been the central paradigm in the field of mental health fifty years ago, this is no longer the case. Biological psychiatry might be viewed as the central paradigm in the mental health field, but there remains a dichotomy between it and the various approaches centered on psychotherapy as the most effective way to remedy emotional disorders such as depression, anxiety, etc. The majority of people seeking psychotherapy describe relationship problems as a central concern. My own view is that most of the conceptual approaches utilized in current psychotherapy remain based on an individualistic paradigm even when couples and families are seen.

It would seem that Bowen theory represents a paradigm in the formal sense of the term. Kuhn wrote that paradigms consist of communities of scholars, investigators, and practitioners who attend the same conferences, share papers, define the problems to be addressed, and train future practitioners. Though knowledge can be shared across paradigms, there are inevitable "translation problems."

The development of Bowen theory has included the integration of knowledge developing in the neurosciences, evolutionary studies, and other natural and social sciences. Beginning in the mid-1970s, the annual symposia sponsored by the Georgetown Family Center included speakers from a wide variety of disciplines in the life sciences. This practice has continued and spread to other Bowen theory centers. This dialogue and the study of knowledge developing in the natural sciences have been the key to the development of the theory. Unique to the theory has been its foundation as a natural systems theory, which is seen as permitting a coherent integration of knowledge across disciplines.

Nevertheless, the basic differences between a systems paradigm and individualistic paradigms create problems in translation. A central aspect of paradigms is that they entail unquestioned belief systems and assumptions which guide the research and its interpretations (Kuhn 2012). The belief systems become institutionalized and thus determine training, hiring, and funding. Interdisciplinary work is more commonplace in the broader fields of science, though it generally occurs within particular paradigms.

Bowen theory, as a natural systems paradigm, is a relatively recent development. The shift to a new paradigm in a given field generally occurs over lengthy periods. There are various factors involved, but often a shift emerges when developing evidence can no longer be reasonably accounted for within an existing paradigm. The "lag time" involved between the introduction of new knowledge and its acceptance in a field or the broader public awareness can range from decades to centuries (Bowen, 2021). The integration of Darwin's theory of evolution into the study of human behavior in psychology is a good example of how long it can take. In addition to apparent "observational blindness," a number of other factors can contribute to the length of time involved, such as significant investments in time and energy by the adherents to a previously accepted paradigm.

In discussing the theory of the family developed by Murray Bowen, it is important to highlight that the term "theory" is used in its formal, scientific sense. As mentioned in chapter 2, his grounding in psychoanalysis at the Menninger Clinic led him to believe that the grounding of that theory in subjectivity prohibited it from moving toward a science of human behavior and becoming integrated with all of science.

Some of the groundwork for a new theory was developed by Bowen while he was still at Menninger's (1945–1954), even though he had not yet considered developing a formal theory to replace psychoanalysis. Bowen's interest in a science of human behavior also contributed to his careful use of terms such as "concepts" and "theory." It led to his view that a science of human behavior would have to be grounded in the facts of evolution if it were to be integrated with the natural sciences. He wrote, "I fashioned a natural systems theory, designed to fit precisely with the principles of evolution and the human as an evolutionary being" (Kerr & Bowen, 1988 p. 360). Given the complexity of family interactions and the number of variables involved, he also believed that a theory of human behavior had to be based on systems thinking.

Following the study at National Institute of Mental Health (NIMH), the development of a new theory later continued at Georgetown University. Bowen wrote that the development of the concept of triangles allowed for the integration of the other concepts into a formal theory of the family which was originally published in the journal *Comprehensive Psychiatry* in 1966 (later reprinted in his 1978 book). The development of this new family systems theory had been decades in the making and included a wide range of concepts and ideas. Bowen described the range of influential ideas that had emerged in writing:

Numerous new ideas emerged from family systems theory. The ideas include (1) *a theory based on facts alone,* (2) *the family diagram,* to handle the voluminous material, (3) *the emotional system,* which included biological facts, in addition to old ideas about feelings, (4) *the differentiation of self,* to denote ways each person is basically different from others, (5) *triangles,* the basic building blocks of any emotional system, carefully separated from the old terms of dyad and triad, (6) *fusion,* to denote ways that people borrow or lend self to another, (7) *cutoffs,* to describe the immature separation of people from each other, (8) *nuclear family emotional system,* to describe the complex ways parents handle emotional process in a single generation, (9) *the nuclear family projection process,* to describe the automatic transmission of problems into future generations, (10) *the extended family emotional system,* to describe unseen involvement of the extended families, (11) *the multigenerational transmission process,* to describe the patterns of emotional process through multiple generations, and (12) *the therapist's involvement of self,* to describe the process through which the therapist becomes involved in the family emotional process, or ways he can be separate from the family unit, (13) the fact that these are all *systems components* of the large emotional system, which is the family, (14) *meshing of the family system with the environment,* to describe the ways the family is part of the total of society. (Kerr & Bowen, 1988 pp. 345–346)

This was a remarkably productive period of conceptual development for Bowen. The development of a new theory went hand in glove with the development of a new form of psychotherapy based on the theory. This occurred in the midst of a larger developing field of family therapy across the country. There was a great deal of excitement related to the emergence of family therapy, but for the most part the importance of theory was obscured. A number of other models of family therapy were also emerging at the time which were highly influential and to varying degrees included forms of systems thinking (Guerin, 1976). Bowen was recognized as a central pioneer in the development of family therapy, while the theory on which the therapy was based received less consideration. The critical importance of shifting from the predominant individualistic paradigm underlying the multitude of psychotherapies at play in the field of mental health was understood by a limited number of clinicians. Family members were increasingly seen in therapy, but "family therapy" was to a great extent seen as a technique to be utilized in intervening with troubled families. Other family systems models were developed underlying family interventions resulting in "schools" of family therapy. Bowen had predicted that without a theory, the various schools would eventually be absorbed by the larger individual-oriented perspective in the field of mental health. After several decades of enthusiastic expansion, the "bloom came off the rose" for the broader family movement as the promise of family therapy for complex human problems fell short of expectations. Lacking a formal theoretical base, in the broader field of mental health, family therapy came to be seen as one of many therapeutic interventions to be considered. Adherents of a family systems paradigm remain, however, as communities of scholars and practitioners engage in a variety of systems conceptual frameworks in defining their practice and research.

The evolutionary biologist David Sloan Wilson (2019) describes a common misunderstanding of theory as it is utilized in science. Theory provides a lens for the observation of natural phenomena. He writes,

> We cannot possibly attend to everything, so a theory—broadly defined as a way of interpreting the world around us—is required to tell us what to pay attention to and what to ignore. We must theorize to see. A new theory doesn't just posit a new interpretation of old observations. It opens doors to new observations to which old theories were blind. (pp. 3–4)

The theory developed by Bowen was based on the classic scientific process of observation, hypothesis development, and hypothesis testing with further observation. When sufficient knowledge about an area of family functioning was attained, a formal concept was constructed. And when a number of interlocking concepts were developed, they constituted a formal theory of the family.

The popular use of the terms theory and concepts can be misleading. In a discussion of the central value of concepts, the evolutionary biologist Ernst Mayr (1982) compared the development of concepts in biology as similar to laws developed in physics, describing "that the history of biology has been dominated by the establishment of concepts and by their maturation, modification, and–occasionally—their rejection" (p. 76).

Even prior to the development of the total theory, Bowen carefully chose concepts based on areas of family functioning that would be consistent with the sciences.

> Early in the research, I made some decisions based on previous thinking about theory. Family research was producing a completely new order of observations. There was a wealth of new theoretical clues. On the premise that psychiatry might eventually become a recognized science, perhaps a generation or two in the future, and being aware of the past conceptual problems of psychoanalysis, I chose to use only concepts that would be consistent with a recognized science. This was done in the hope that investigators of the future would more easily be able to see connections between human behavior and the accepted sciences than we can. I therefore chose to use concepts that would be consistent with biology and the natural sciences. (Bowen, 1978 p. 354)

Bowen theory provided a new way of viewing human behavior which had not been previously seen. The older and still common individualistic paradigm, I believe, has contributed to the observational blindness. This paradigm entails seeing families as social groups shaped primarily by social norms and made up of varying personalities as opposed to being highly integrated, interdependent living systems. Behavior is seen as emanating from individuals who may have been shaped by their genes, their families, or their cultures. Bowen theory is distinct in viewing the family as a natural system which functions as a self-regulating system and whose members are continuously influencing each other in a largely automatic and patterned manner.

The theory "opens the door" to viewing the family emotional system. It is a systems theory and its eight interlocking concepts provide a conceptual framework which can allow one to see the underlying oneness at play in all families. Each concept describes elements of family functioning, but they are interrelated and need to be seen in the context of the whole theory. I apologize for some redundancy, as a number of the concepts have been discussed in previous chapters, but I think the presentation of the theory as a whole might be useful. In this chapter, I will briefly describe the eight concepts and hopefully to some degree capture how each is interrelated to the others and to the theory as a whole. The exercise of considering all the concepts in observing a family can contribute to systems thinking and provide a way of overcoming the observational blindness entailed in individualistic thinking.

The integration of the various concepts into a systems theory is based on the proposition that the family is an emotional system. Bowen (1978) writes,

> Some background about the theory will help in understanding the separate concepts. This is a theory about the functioning of the emotional system in man. In broad terms, the *emotional system* is conceived to be the function of the life forces inherited from his phylogenetic past, that he shares with the lower forms, and that governs the subhuman part of man. It would be synonymous with instinct, if instinct is considered to include forces that operate automatically. . . . This theory postulates that more of man's life and behavior is governed by automatic emotional forces than he can easily admit. (p. 423)

All of the concepts refer to the automatic emotional processes at play in the human family. The concept of differentiation of self describes an automatic developmental process occurring in the context of the family relationship system. It also entails the degree to which an individual attains the capacity to have some choice. While all of the concepts in Bowen theory refer to automatic processes involved in behavior, the expression of the concepts in the functioning of families and individuals is influenced by the level of maturity or differentiation involved. It is an interesting exercise to consider how the expression of each of the seven other concepts in a family will vary based on this central concept.

NUCLEAR FAMILY EMOTIONAL PROCESS

This concept describes the observable interactional patterns occurring in each nuclear family described in chapter 4: emotional distance in the marital pair; conflict in their relationship; the reciprocal over- and under-functioning in the marriage; and the involvement of a child in the fusion of the marital pair. The patterns are principally affected by the level of differentiation of self and the amount of stress a family is contending with. The patterns are most easily observable during periods of heightened stress. They represent mechanisms families utilize to adapt to the level of their fusion or oneness.

The greater the level of fusion among members in a family unit, the more their thoughts, feelings, and behavior are determined by their reactions to one another. The more fused, the more sensitized members are to each other, and the more other-directed than self-directed their behavior is. During a family's more stressful times, an increase in tension or chronic anxiety occurs. In response, there is an instinctual "pulling together" among members, which is adaptive in the short term, but creates problems when prolonged over time. For those functioning at lower levels of differentiation, the pulling together can, over time, be experienced as threatening. The emotional sensitivity members have with one another can result in one member distancing as a way to decrease their anxiety or tension, while another experiences the distance as a threat to their relationship. Each is responding to the other and can result in an escalation in their emotional reactivity. The four nuclear family mechanisms occur automatically and typically result with an increase in either blaming oneself for the increased tension or blaming the other.

In addition to differentiation of self and the level of chronic anxiety, the extent to which a nuclear family is isolated from the larger extended family is a major factor in contributing to the emotional intensity operating in a family. When family members can be in better contact with the larger family, the family's adaptive capacity is enhanced. When isolated, the underlying emotional dependence members have on one another becomes more exaggerated under stress. Members will either experience more pressure from the others to "be for them" or pressure the others to "be for self" to alleviate their own stress or uncertainty. The isolation of a family can result in an increase in a family's fusion or oneness resulting in greater emotional reactivity in the unit.

While members in all family units will react to one another during stressful times, those families which function at higher levels of differentiation will utilize the family mechanisms to a lesser degree. Individuals evidencing more self have a greater capacity to tolerate increases in tension in others and in self and as a result will react less automatically to others during stressful periods. They may initially react automatically when they or another family member are stressed, but in having a greater capacity to regulate their emotional reactivity, they have an ability to respond more thoughtfully. As Bowen writes: "This concept describes the pattern of emotional forces as they operate over the years in the nuclear family" (Bowen, 1978 p. 425).

In addition to differentiation of self, the other six concepts in the theory also influence the expression of the nuclear family emotional process. For example, the birth order of each member will have an influence on how each family member participates in the process (Toman, 1969). The family projection process, triangles, and the multigenerational transmission process influence the expression and degree of a family's adaptive mechanisms. In addition, the extent to which a nuclear family is cut off from the larger extended family and is influenced by the societal emotional process also are factors at play. The inclusion of the interlocking eight concepts of the theory in the study of families contributes to the observation of the system and how it functions.

NUCLEAR FAMILY PROJECTION PROCESS

Bowen defined one of the nuclear family adaptive mechanisms as a separate concept due to its importance in the total theory. Each family and its members must adapt to their position in the family and the family's position in the multigenerational family in addition to the larger environment. As mentioned in chapter 4, there is variation among offspring in the degree to which they develop or mature. This involves separating out from the family oneness and the development of a self.

The concept of the family projection process describes the greater involvement of one child in the parental fusion than the others. In this process, the parents project some of their own immaturity to one or more of their children. It is an active process in which parental anxiety is alleviated in their relationship by a focus on or concern about one of their children. The concern or anxiety about one child more than the others can be initially triggered by real events such as a premature birth requiring a prolonged hospitalization or a physical defect requiring surgery. But the concern develops into a functional process when the heightened emotional involvement continues after the initial difficulties have passed. It becomes a functional process when the anxiety resulting from the fusion in the marital pair is directed toward the child. The parental overinvolvement with a child, however, does not require a reality-based concern. A child may be selected for the projection process due to being the first-born, the first of a given sex, or the youngest. It may be principally due to the pregnancy and birth occurring during an especially difficult period for the family, such as the death of a family member.

The parental focus on a child can be expressed in many ways. In general, it principally involves the mother, with the father or other principal caretaker in a supportive role. It can take the form of seeing the child as more fragile or as more difficult. It can be the one mother "falls in love with." While mother may be the one most emotionally involved with a child, the family projection process involves more than the mother. As Kerr (2019) writes,

> The concept describes a mechanism for how anxiety gets transmitted from a parent to a developing child. It is important to remember here that the level of chronic anxiety in a mother is not simply a property of the mother. Her level of anxiety reflects the level of anxiety in the family system of which she is a part and the larger network of relationships in which the family system exists, such as the extended family and community. (p. 105)

It can be difficult for many to recognize that loving parental care as well as abusive parental care can equally contribute to constraining the development of a child. When viewed from the perspective of the family as a unit, and when a family can be observed going through its most stressful times, the projection process can more easily be seen as having a stabilizing function for the unit. The "love" for one child may entail a level of emotional involvement which can inhibit the development of emotional autonomy for that child. It is a process occurring to greater or lesser degrees in all families and it is not whether the parental emotional involvement is positive or negative but the level of fusion that exists in the parental triangle. Bowen defined the family projection process as a separate concept as it "describes the most important way family emotional process is transmitted from one generation to the next" (Bowen, 1978 p. 425).

The family projection process also needs to be seen in the context of the other concepts as each is involved in this family pattern. Each aspect of family functioning defined in the other seven concepts plays a part in the family projection process. It is not easy for most people to come to grips with the idea that as a parent one can contribute to constricting the development of one of their children. What could be further from the intention of a parent? A parent may blame their spouse for their child's difficulties or blame themselves. The blaming often takes the form of either one parent not having done enough or having harmed the child by being overly strict or lenient. Or both parents may blame the child whose difficulties were due to a variety of reasons. A child, whose parents have been especially concerned about his behavior, may raise mayhem during adolescence. The parental focus which may have been there all along is now centered on what is perceived as rebelliousness and lack of consideration for the parents.

A very different view emerges when a motivated parent can gain some objectivity about the automaticity involved in the family projection process, when they can begin to acknowledge the part they may have played but also come to see that part in the broader context of the family emotional system. The projection process is a triangle set in the multigenerational family process as well as in the events and environmental stressors contributing to the chronic anxiety at play in the family. Each member of the triangle as well as other members play a part but do not cause the process. When some objectivity can be attained, blaming recedes. And when one member can recognize a part they play in the process, it creates the potential for them to begin to modify their part. When a parent can begin to take some responsibility and begin to define themselves more clearly in the marital relationship, some of the focus on a child can begin to lessen. Parents do not choose to focus on one of their children. It is an automatic adaptive process. Once the projection process can be observed in the context of the other family concepts, it becomes easier to see the bind that each member of the triangle is caught up in.

TRIANGLES

The family projection process is a form of what Bowen defined as a triangle. He used the term "triangle" to distinguish it from the term he used early in the NIMH study in which he described the father, mother, and schizophrenic adult child as the *interdependent triad* (Bowen, 1978 p. 26). He substituted "triangle" in order to convey the fluid process occurring among three people. As Bowen was working on his theory of the family in the mid-1960s, it was his work on the concept of triangles that "was the cement that integrated the concepts into a single theory" (Kerr & Bowen, 1988 p. 379).

Bowen had observed that two-person relationships were basically unstable in that they will predictably involve a third person when tension inevitably arises. When tension does arise in the original twosome, one of the two will involve a third person either by talking about the other, or by distancing and "joining" with the third person. This involvement of another serves the function of decreasing the original tension. The third person may either side with one or distance in order to not take sides. If the outside third-party distances, the recruitment of another third party typically takes place. If the tension continues to increase in this initial triangle, another person will be involved leading to what Bowen described as interlocking triangles.

Triangles are usually in a constant state of motion as individuals move to be on the inside with another, seek to move to the outside, or are extruded to the outside. Bowen described triangles as the building blocks of all relationship systems, family, or otherwise. In periods of higher tension or stress, the triangles are most observable, though not usually to those within them. They are basic to behavior and so automatic that for the most part they operate outside of awareness. It is a property of all relationship systems and predictable that when an organization goes through a more difficult time, the level of triangling in the form of gossip will increase. An individual will seek to become comfortable by moving toward another and relieving their tension by talking about the "problem" other. The other may welcome the contact initially, but as the tension is unloaded, he or she will either take sides against a third or "remember" a meeting they had to go to.

In the family, for example, a mother and daughter may have a conflict resulting in mother later going to her spouse with her report. Father may side with her and later go to daughter to scold her or commiserate about mother's bad mood. If he gets into conflict with daughter, mother may then criticize his parenting and side with her daughter. The range of triangle patterns are numerous, though they become quite predictable in individual families.

Triangles have an important function in relationship systems as they serve to decrease tension for some. In a 1976 interview, Bowen stated that

> a "triangle" is a "natural way of being" for people. . . . The two person relationship is unstable in that it has a low tolerance for anxiety and it is easily disturbed by emotional forces within the twosome and by relationship forces from outside the twosome. . . . With involvement of the third person, the anxiety level decreases. It is as if the anxiety is diluted as it shifts from one person to another of the three relationships in a triangle. The triangle is more stable and flexible than the twosome. It has a much higher tolerance for anxiety and is capable of handling a fair percentage of life stresses. (Bowen, 1978 p. 400)

With enough intensity, however, the triangling process can result in a family member absorbing sufficient tension to result in the development of symptoms (Klever, 2009). In the workplace it can result in an employee being fired. Knowledge of triangles, on the other hand, can allow a motivated family member or an influential member of an organization to interrupt the flow of anxiety by not distancing or taking sides while remained engaged with both. The triangle is also central to the psychotherapy based on Bowen theory. More will be discussed about this in the next chapter.

MULTIGENERATIONAL TRANSMISSION PROCESS

It can be said that to some degree each of us is born into a central triangle. For most, this consists of ourselves and our parents. In some families it may be one's mother and maternal grandmother when, for example, the father is absent. In previous centuries when the incidence of the death of mothers during childbirth was high, the triangle might include father and a member of his family or the child might be adopted by one of the parents' siblings and their spouse. But it is rare to find an isolated dyad consisting only of one caretaker and a child. When that is the case, the emotional separation between mother and child, so important to the development of adaptive capacity, will be greatly impaired.

It can also be said that each sibling is born into and develops in a different triangle. The parents may be the same, but the triangle will to some degree function differently based on a number of factors such as the birth order and sex of a child or changes in the larger family configuration or environment occurring around the birth of a child. Even though siblings develop in the same family, their functional positions and course of development will vary to some degree. And this phenotypic variation among siblings is writ large over the generations of a family.

The concept of the multigenerational transmission process, described in chapter 7, appears to have had its initial beginnings by Bowen during the NIMH research study in which he came to the conclusion that schizophrenia was not likely to develop in just one or two generations. The observation of the nuclear family emotional process and the projection of parental immaturity to a child in the research families indicated that similar processes existed in the parents' families of origin. His later detailed study of a few families, including his own, demonstrated that the patterns could be observed to occur in each generation and that the process, over multiple generations, would lead to the maximum impairment of an offspring. Variation in the overall functioning of siblings in each generation constituted a process generating a wide range of functioning among the descendants of an original family.

The concept of the multigenerational transmission process, similar to the others in the theory, is not a stand-alone concept. In addition to requiring a significant amount of factual information about a family's history, the observation of this process also involves knowledge of the theory's other seven concepts. With sufficient facts of the nuclear families in several proceeding generations, it is possible to discern emotional patterns operating in each generation and how the functioning of each family is shaped by its previous generations and shapes the functioning of succeeding generations (Klever, 2015).

EMOTIONAL CUTOFF

The evolution of the highly interdependent human family entailing a prolonged period of development for offspring created a dilemma for all its members: how to manage their remaining level of unresolved emotional attachment. Bowen developed the concept of emotional cutoff to describe the principal mechanism utilized by individuals as each generation seeks to separate from the parental generation. The greater the emotional dependence, the greater difficulty individuals have in establishing themselves in the next generation. It is part of a multigenerational process in that each generation is influenced by the level of emotional cutoff the parents established with their own parents.

Each generation is faced with the task of moving into adulthood while remaining to some degree emotionally dependent on the parental family. The level of remaining emotional dependence was referred to by Bowen as the degree of "unresolved emotional attachment." He described this unresolved attachment in writing:

It is necessary to think of all degrees of unresolved emotional attachment. The most differentiated people are those with fairly differentiated parents. They have been more free to grow away from parents since childhood. When they reach adolescence there is less attachment against which they have to struggle. Physical maturation and growing toward the responsibilities of adult life is more of a challenge than a struggle with the parents. The degree of emotional turmoil at adolescence is one good indicator of the unresolved emotional attachment. Some degree of adolescent rebellion is so common it is considered by many to be a "normal" stage in life. A fairly well differentiated person has comparatively less unresolved emotional attachment to the parental family. The move to a self-sustaining life away from the parental family in young adulthood is smoother. More differentiated people have more emotional autonomy within themselves, and more choice of living close to the parents or living far away. The physical proximity to the parents is governed more by reality than by the degree of emotional attachment. (Bowen, 2017 p. 54)

Emotional cutoff is a universal phenomenon, though its expression may appear differently in different cultures. The emotional distancing between the generations can be intrapsychic or geographic. In a collectivistic culture, for example, individuals may more likely retain close contact with the parents, but the unresolved emotional attachment will be evidenced by less openness in their relationships. An individual may appear to have attained more emotional autonomy in an individualistic culture when he or she has minimal contact with parents, but the unresolved attachment and resulting cut off will also be more apparent in the degree of openness existing in the relationships. By itself, geographic closeness or distance is not an indicator of the degree of existing emotional cutoff. Cutting off is largely automatic and generally operates out of awareness. It can provide an important function in allowing individuals to move forward in their lives, though it also entails some cost. As Kerr writes,

> Bowen theory does not assert that people should not cut off from their families; it says that this is what people do and that it has its advantages and disadvantages. The principal advantage is that it can provide some peace from difficult and painful interactions with one's family; the principal disadvantage is that it intensifies future relationships and the problems associated with an even more anxiety-driven fusion. (Kerr, 2019 p. 144)

The more exaggerated and overt forms of cutoff can be observed in everyone's multigenerational history. It is an important concept which both informs and is informed by the other concepts in the theory. Developing the ability to recognize emotional cutoff in one's own family represents an important element in the effort to become more knowledgeable about one's family and how one functions in emotionally important relationships.

SIBLING POSITION

As mentioned, one of Murray Bowen's objectives in developing a theory of human behavior was to minimize as much subjectivity in it as possible. The sibling position of an individual is a fact. How much does knowledge of an individual's sibling position contribute to knowledge about his or her behavior? To his or her functioning in relationship systems? Bowen's study of the family led him to see it as an important variable and needed to be included in the theory. When he came across the work of Austrian psychologist Walter Toman, he found it to be consistent with his own observations and so decided to include it in the theory.

In his book *Family Constellation* (1969), Toman wrote,

> The purpose of this book is to describe the most important and most easily distinguishable effects of various different social and family environments. We proceed from the assumption that a person's family represents the most influential context of his life, and that it exerts its influence more regularly, more exclusively, and earlier in a person's life than do any other life contexts. (p. 5)

Toman's research was based on the simple premise, then, that one's earliest relationships will influence later life relationships. The day in and day out interactions with siblings is a major element occurring throughout development. The only child is also influenced by his or her position in the family. In his research on sibling position, Toman principally looked at two variables: rank (oldest, middle, youngest) and sex (male, female). He developed eleven sibling profiles based on these variables (oldest brother of brothers, oldest sister of brothers, youngest brother of sisters, etc.).

One's sibling position is a fact. Toman consistently used the expression "all things being equal" to note that other variables are at play which will influence how one's sibling position is expressed in relationship interactions and personality. Like most concepts in biology, it is a probabilistic concept that has a good deal of predictability. When taken into account, the other concepts in Bowen theory contribute to how an individual's sibling position might vary from Toman's profile. For example, an oldest son may function more as a youngest child if he is the object of the family projection process. The development of his maturity may be more constricted, and the next or other sibling may assume the function of an oldest son.

I have thought of the concept as analogously entailing a "position effect," which in genetics refers to how the expression of a gene changes when its location in a chromosome is changed. "All things being equal" the position one is born into will influence the functioning of that person for life. The profiles Toman developed refer to both personality characteristics and how people behave in relationship to others. One's birth order refers to how one influences others and how one is influenced by them. In family research, it is evident that the birth orders of a marital pair are a major influence on the relationship. In family therapy it is often striking how consideration of this variable can change the partners' view of one another.

When I was first exposed to the concept, I was somewhat skeptical of its importance. I could find all the exceptions. Experience with more clinical families, surveying the research literature on the subject of sibling position, and the study of my own family, led me to see its importance in understanding behavior. I still recall an early clinical example which highlighted the impact of sibling position on relationships.

I met with a couple who had been married for twelve years. It was an initial session in which each expressed their dissatisfaction with their relationship. They spoke of an increasing emotional distance and frustration. Neither expressed much hope for change and by the end of the session, I also thought the therapy most likely was not going to go anywhere. In looking at their family diagram, I noticed that they were both the youngest in their families of origin. Without much hope that either was sufficiently motivated to initiate any change, I tossed out a comment about their sibling positions and briefly described Toman's profiles along with how their sibling position may or may not be an influence on their relationship. We scheduled another appointment, which I suspected they would likely cancel in the coming week.

Much to my surprise, they returned and were quite animated in discussing how they thought their sibling positions played a major part in their disaffection. They described that from their early courtship days on, each had looked to the other to take initiative around decisions large and small. In considering their positions as a youngest in their families, they said they had begun to see how they each contributed to the paralysis they experienced with one another. Their views changed from seeing the other as weak or passive to a clearer understanding of the expectations each had of the other and their own roles in the marriage. This slight increase in objectivity allowed them to not take the other's indecisiveness so personally. It also led them to be more curious about what other factors might be influencing their relationship. Needless to say, it increased my own interest in exploring the influence of sibling position.

The concept of sibling position provides one with a valuable lens for exploring the functioning of individuals and relationships among family members. Seen in the context of the multigenerational family, in addition to the marital relationship, it raises questions about one's parents and their relationship with each child. Knowledge of an individual's sibling position has the potential to add some objectivity to the study of the family and its members. In discussing the subject of parenting Toman (1969) wrote,

> The influence that their (the parents) sibling roles and their compatibility with each other as well as with the configuration of their children exert on their family life and on their children's psychological and social development is only a portion of their total influence. Yet it can be more easily observed and objectively and systematically described than other influences emanating from the parents. (pp. 198–199)

While sibling position is only a portion of an individual's functioning, the other seven concepts in Bowen theory contribute to how it might fit in the total family and influence an individual's personality and relationship functioning.

SOCIETAL EMOTIONAL PROCESS

Murray Bowen was invited by the Environmental Protection Agency to present a paper at a 1972 symposium on the environmental crisis. He was asked to present on the subject of predictable human reactions to crises. The invitation encouraged him to devote his thinking to a subject which had been of interest to him for many years—the interplay between emotional process in the family and emotional process in society. Over the next several years, he refined his thinking on the topic and in 1976 he introduced it as the eighth concept in Bowen theory.

The concept is based on the view that the human is a biological, instinctual creature and that emotional process governs much of human behavior at the societal level as it does in the family. In 1974, Bowen presented a paper at a memorial conference for the pioneering family therapist Nathan Ackerman entitled "Societal Regression as Viewed through Family Systems Theory." In the paper, he described what he saw as a period of societal regression occurring in the United States with characteristics similar to regressions occurring in families. Bowen saw regressions as occurring in response to increases in chronic anxiety and a resulting loss in the functional level of differentiation at the societal level. In a family, regression proceeds when decisions are made to alleviate the current anxiety rather than address the underlying sources of the anxiety. Parents can avoid making difficult or principled decisions which might upset a child or spouse. This may reduce the tension of the moment but further invites greater anxiety when the issues arise again. Decisions are made based on a feeling response rather than on a thoughtful, principled basis.

A similar process was seen by Bowen as occurring at the societal level when leadership and legislative decisions were made to apply band-aid approaches to underlying problems and the avoidance of difficult decisions. He came to see that the underlying chronic anxiety evident in society was a result of the human's instinctive awareness of a growing disharmony between man and nature. Regarding the regression that he observed, he wrote,

> The hypothesis postulates that man's increasing anxiety is a product of population explosion, the disappearance of new habitable land to colonize, the approaching depletion of raw materials necessary to sustain life, and growing awareness that "spaceship earth" cannot indefinitely support human life in the style to which man and his technology have become accustomed. (Bowen, 1978 p. 272)

Bowen changed the term "societal regression" to "societal emotional process" for this concept due to the view that historically societies go through periods of progression as well as regression. It also appeared that both processes could be occurring simultaneously with some segments of society undertaking actions which are regressive, while others might be progressing. He did, however, see current society as going through a sustained regression and that, similar to families in a regression, would only shift when the distress created by the regression was greater than the pain required to adequately reverse its course.

Michael Kerr (2019) aptly describes characteristics of a societal regression:

> The fundamental process at work in emotional regressions is that principle-determined decisions and actions give way to a more feeling orientation. This happens in the family, and it happens in the larger society. Other manifestations of this shift from principle to feeling include a rising incidence of violence, with much of it being domestic violence, as well as more we-they factions characterized by extreme self-righteousness, rapid changes in mores (these changes are considered regressive because a more pressured feeling orientation replaces a more rational and contemplative process), less stable intimate relationships with overall higher divorce rates (this can fluctuate over time), more focus on rights than responsibilities, more crime, more litigation, more substance abuse, a rise in teen pregnancies, permissiveness, radical dogmatic fundamentalism, a more pervasive attitude of entitlement, less responsibility for the environment, quick-fix legislation to relieve the anxiety of the moment, omnipresence of conspiracy theories, and a rise in terrorism. (p. 156)

Bowen observed another pattern occurring at the societal level that is similar to one observable in the family: that of the family projection process. At the family level, an increase in the level of chronic anxiety can result in a more exaggerated focus on a child who is believed to be more vulnerable or problematic. The increased focus on a child by the family can take the form of an overly sympathetic response to a perceived frailty or "weakness" or an overly harsh, punitive response to the perceived negative behavior of the child. Each family member in varying degrees, including the focused upon child, are active participants in this process. This can serve as a stabilizing process for the family, despite the loss of functioning or impairment in an individual child.

The projection process at the societal level generally takes the form of a projection onto a minority population. Similar to the family process, a group can be perceived to be problematic or even as a threat, or as more fragile and less capable. Both an overly sympathetic or overly harsh projection can result in the loss of functioning of the members of such a group. The necessary constructive responses to the sources of a society's chronic anxiety, be it climate change, over-population, or decreasing economic opportunities, are neglected as a particular population is seen as "the problem" to be addressed.

It is not difficult to see how a society, such as our current one, can contribute to difficulties families will have in their functioning. Families at lower levels of differentiation will be more greatly affected by the societal emotional process, while those at higher levels will have a greater capacity to withstand societal pressures and remain more on course. Families are not immune to societal emotional process and the concept provides a link to the social environment in which a family exists. It is difficult for most to see the human as an instinctual, evolutionary creature. The concept of societal emotional process highlights how interdependent the human is with nature as well as the degree to which the family is influenced by the larger societal processes.

Despite the potential the human has to use intellect to solve complex problems, Murray Bowen was not optimistic about the short-term adaptiveness of Homo sapiens. He prophetically wrote,

> If my hypothesis about societal anxiety is reasonably accurate, the crises of society will recur and recur, with increasing intensity for decades to come. Man created the environmental crisis by being the kind of creature he is. The environment is part of man, change will require a change in the basic nature of man, and man's track record for that kind of change has not been good. Man is a versatile animal and perhaps he will be able to change faster when confronted with the alternatives. I believe man is moving into crises of unparalleled

proportions, that the crises will be different than those he has faced before, that they will come with increasing frequency for several decades, that he will go as far as he can in dealing symptomatically with each crisis, and that a final major crisis will come as soon as the middle of the next century. The type of man who survives that will be one who can live in better harmony with nature. (Bowen, 1978, p. 281)

DIFFERENTIATION OF SELF

Genetic inheritance alone would insure the uniqueness of each individual and variation in their adaptive capacity. The contribution of genetic material from each parent results in a unique genotype for individuals in the next generation. The interaction of this genotype with the environment results in the further uniqueness, resulting in the fact that in Homo sapiens' 300,000 year presence on planet Earth, there has never existed someone exactly like you; nor will there ever be again.

The recently burgeoning field of epigenetics has greatly expanded our understanding of inheritance and how the experience of the previous generations might influence the expression or silencing of genes contributing to individual differences and variation in adaptive capacity. Among the transgenerational epigenetic processes affecting individual differences of offspring are those shaping the reactivity to stress (Meaney, 2010) and parental care (Champagne, 2008).

Based on a series of pioneering research studies, Michael Meaney's lab at McGill University not only demonstrated the epigenetic transmission of traits over multiple generations but discovered the neural and molecular substrates involved. In a 2004 paper they write,

> Our findings provide the first evidence that maternal behavior produces stable alterations of DNA methylation and chromatin structure, providing a mechanism for the long-term effects of maternal care on gene expression in offspring. (Weaver et al., 2004 p. 852)

Another discovery of gene–environment interactions shaping individual variation was the discovery of genetic polymorphisms. Polymorphisms occur when two versions of the same gene, one from each parent, exist at the same site on a chromosome. One such polymorphism has been found to influence an offspring's responsiveness to either more positive or adverse environments. Variation in this responsiveness results in offspring that are biologically sensitive to their environmental context (Boyce & Ellis, 2005). It has been posited that the existence of such polymorphisms may have been selected for due to their adaptive value allowing some offspring to take advantage of a more stable environment or more reactive to stress in a more threatening environment (Ellis et al. 2011).

The emergence of another field of study called "human social genomics" has further eroded the nature/nurture dichotomy in discovering the existence of many genes that are regulated by social-environmental signals. George Slavich and Steven Cole at UCLA describe what they have termed the "biological embedding of social experience" (2013). Recent discoveries have demonstrated the ongoing influence of the social environment on gene expression. The neural and molecular mechanisms involved have been elucidated in how adverse conditions can contribute to vulnerability to disease. They write,

> Although additional research is needed to evaluate how widespread and deep the effects of social adversity on gene expression are, the fact that social influences can remodel transcriptional activity in the brain (and not just in the periphery of the body) is particularly important because it provides a biologically plausible explanation for how social adversity may elicit the wide range of neural, psychological, and behavioral alterations that characterize mental and physical health problems that have been associated with adverse social-environmental circumstances. (Slavich & Cole, 2013 p. 335)

The above epigenetic research has greatly expanded our knowledge of the biological and social factors contributing to the development of individual differences in adaptive capacity. Tie-Yuan Zhang and Michael Meaney (2005) describe this phenomenon in writing:

> Indeed, maternal effects could result in the transmission of adaptive responses across generations. In humans, such effects might contribute to the familial transmission of risk and resilience. Finally, it is interesting to consider the possibility that epigenetic changes could be an intermediate process that imprints dynamic environmental experiences on the fixed genome, resulting in stable alterations in phenotype—a process of environment-dependent chromatin plasticity. (p. 462)

Murray Bowen's research and his development of Bowen theory have contributed to this knowledge by the inclusion of the human family in understanding the development of individual differences in adaptive capacity. The concepts of the emotional system and differentiation of self provide a conceptual framework for the integration of this emerging knowledge. Bowen's description of the self as "composed of constitutional, physical, physiological, biological, genetic and cellular reactivity factors, as they move in unison with psychological factors" (Kerr & Bowen, 1988 p. 342) captures the reciprocal signaling at play among an individual's biological and psychological systems. The focus on the family as the unit of study added another level of complexity and defined its role as a regulatory system involving its components.

As mentioned in chapter 3, the concept of differentiation of self describes how individuals vary in their basic adaptiveness. Bowen observed that individuals differ in the degree of differentiation of their emotional and intellectual systems, a process occurring in the context of the family over the course of development. Based on this observation, he developed a continuum along which all people could be placed, from the lowest levels of adaptive capacity to the potentially highest levels. At the lowest levels, people's lives are governed by the automatic emotional system and they have little capacity to chart their own course in life. They are almost totally at the mercy of their relationship environment. Upon reaching late adolescence or young adulthood, they have great difficulty in managing their functioning apart from the family. Faced with the challenges of adulthood, they are vulnerable to the development of psychiatric, physical, or behavioral symptoms. The lack of differentiation of their intellectual system leaves them with little ability to navigate a course for themselves and many can live out their lives either in isolation or dependent on their family or institutions. This is a small percentage of the human population and they can be found across cultures. It is important to note that this is not a category of individuals but simply the lowest level on a continuum of human adaptation.

A bit higher up on the continuum of differentiation are those individuals whose lives remain largely relationship dependent, but they have a greater capacity to move forward in their lives when the environment is more favorable or stable. They can think for themselves in areas not involving important relationships and when the stressors in their lives are minimal. In their important relationships they are highly sensitive to how they are viewed and to the functioning of those on whom they are most dependent. When their relationship system is disturbed, they are more vulnerable to the development of symptoms or to dependently over-functioning for another family member. They are more likely to be compliant or emotionally reactive, managing their dependence on others with ongoing relationship patterns of distance, conflict, or symptomatic behavior. Their life energy is directed toward seeking approval or love with little left for developing and pursuing their own life goals. At this level of differentiation their lives are more feeling-oriented and the seeking of comfort and avoidance of discomfort remain central.

The lives of individuals at a more moderate level of differentiation have a little more capacity to use their thinking or intellectual system in directing their lives. They may be relationship-oriented but have more flexibility in how they respond to life challenges or emotional stimuli. They may still be vulnerable to symptom development when sufficiently stressed, but the symptoms are less pronounced or prolonged. They remain sensitive to the reactions of others, but their own behavior is not totally determined by the approval or emotional states of others in their relationship systems. In short, they have some capacity to think for themselves. They may lose that ability when stress is running high in the family or work systems, but they are able to retain it when the tension subsides. People at more moderate levels of differentiation have more life energy to pursue goals for themselves, though they have difficulty in sustaining a direction when they or their relationship system is significantly disturbed. There is greater awareness of how the automatic emotional system can at times be problematic for them, and they may muster enough discipline to pursue a course of action which assists in managing themselves more effectively during heightened periods of stress.

As mentioned, the concept of differentiation of self entails differences among individuals in the degree of differentiation between the feeling and intellectual systems. Those higher on the continuum have a greater capacity to utilize their intellectual system in directing their life course. A brief quote by Bowen (1978) characterizes how this is manifested in their lives.

> Those in the upper part of this group (individuals with moderate to good levels of differentiation of self) are those in which there is more solid self. Persons with a functional intellectual system are no longer a prisoner of the emotional-feeling world. They are able to live life more freely and to have more satisfying emotional lives within the emotional system. They can participate fully in emotional events knowing that they can extricate themselves with logical reasoning when the need arises. There may be periods of laxness in which they permit the automatic pilot of the emotional system to have full control, but when trouble develops they can take over, calm the anxiety, and avoid a life crisis. People with better levels of differentiation are less relationship directed and more able to follow independent life goals. They are not unaware of the relationship system, but their life courses can be determined more from within themselves than from what others think. They are more clear about the differences between emotion and intellect, and they are better able to state their own convictions and beliefs calmly without attacking the beliefs of others or without having to defend their own. They are better able to accurately evaluate themselves in relation to others without the pretend postures that result in overvaluing or undervaluing themselves (pp. 369–370).

The concept of differentiation of self is central to Bowen theory and influences how the other seven concepts are expressed in a family. It defines the adaptive capacity of individuals and families in a rich and expanded manner.

The concept posits that the family is the principal source of variation found among individuals in their adaptive capacity. It also defines the developmental process involved in the differentiation of higher cortical systems (the intellectual system) as central to adaptive capacity.

Each of the eight concepts in Bowen theory describes aspects of family functioning. As an interrelated whole they provide a conceptual framework for systems thinking. Science and the future will determine how accurate this theory is. The development of the theory by Bowen is an applicable one, providing people with a framework for the study of their own functioning and that of their families. And in doing so it also entails a way for people to increase their adaptive capacity and contribute to the functioning of their families.

Chapter 10

Family as a Pathway toward Enhancing Adaptive Capacity

The observation that the family functions as an emotional system, that it maintains a relatively stable oneness over time, led to the observation that individual members vary in the degree to which they adhere to one another, the degree to which they have or have not attained a basic level of self over the course of their development. Families vary in the degree of their oneness or their "undifferentiated ego mass" as Bowen once described it. Bowen used that term in an effort to describe a family's oneness to those in the field of psychiatry and in later years rarely used the term. In describing the "family ego mass" Bowen (1978) writes,

> Theoretically, a family ego mass can be considered to include the members of the nuclear family, father-mother-children, and to extend back into the extended family network to include all members of the extended families who still have unresolved emotional dependencies on each other. (p. 113)

The term "undifferentiated ego mass" does, however, capture the degree of oneness or togetherness operating in a family system and the degree to which individuals have not attained an emotionally autonomous self. The greater the undifferentiation in a family the more a member's functioning is regulated by the family relationship system than it is by self. The greater the undifferentiation in a family, the less adaptive capacity the family and its members will have.

Psychotherapy with families provided Bowen with an observational perch which allowed him to observe the togetherness processes at play in a family when a member undertook an effort to be more of a self, to operate more out of self. Such an effort highlights a family's emotional equilibrium and the effort to maintain it in response to a member's attempt to be less fused.

Family members involved in the family ego mass are bogged down in an emotional morass of interdependence, each too dependent on the other to risk becoming a clear self. Spouses become so involved in being the way the other wants them to be to improve the functioning of the other, and demanding that the other be different to enhance the functioning of self, that neither is responsible for self. When either spouse is able to define and maintain a definite identity from this amorphous feeling mass, the first step in the recovery process is underway. This involves maintaining a self in the face of emotional pressure from the other, and maintaining responsibility for self without so much emotional demand on the other. (Bowen, 1978 p. 114)

Bowen theory, and its concepts of the emotional system and differentiation of self, provides a new lens for observing ourselves and for options in modifying our behavior. It includes the observation that we are embedded in a family emotional process shaping our behavior which is largely automatic and operating outside of awareness. It is possible to observe this process, predict its operation, and then have some choice in how to respond. It includes the potential for increasing the level of one's functioning and the capacity to adapt to life challenges.

It is not my intention to describe in any detail the application of Bowen theory in psychotherapy. That would be the subject of a book in itself and aspects of the theory's application can be found in other publications (Bowen, 1978; Kerr, 2019; Kerr & Bowen, 1988; Papero, 1990). Fundamentally, the application of Bowen theory in psychotherapy requires a grounding in the theory and the development of the ability to think systems (Kerr, 2019). It also requires an effort on the part of the clinician to undertake both the study of one's own family and to define oneself in relation to the family and important others. In describing the objective of psychotherapy based on Bowen theory, Bowen (1978) wrote,

The therapy based on differentiation is no longer therapy in the usual sense. The therapy is as different from conventional therapy as the theory is different from conventional theory. The over-all goal is to help individual family members to rise up out of the emotional togetherness that binds us all. (p. 371)

In this chapter, I would like to present an approach developed by Bowen allowing individuals to undertake such an effort. It is an effort to increase one's level of functioning, to "rise up" a bit, and to increase one's ability to think systems.

The development of the family systems theory by Murray Bowen went hand in glove with the development of a clinical approach. During the period of his involvement at the Menninger Foundation, he was formally trained in psychoanalytic theory and psychotherapy. As I mentioned in chapter 9,

Bowen's interest in contributing to a science of human behavior led him to have many questions about that theory and its application. He became curious about the impact parents had on the residential patients at the clinic when they would visit their sons or daughters.

Though it was heretical in psychoanalytical circles at the time to meet with the families of the patients being treated by psychiatrists, Bowen began to meet with the families during their weekend visits. This resulted in his making observations which were markedly different than those viewed through the lens of psychoanalytic theory (Bowen, 2013a; Kerr, 2020). He could observe the dramatic impact the families, and especially the mothers, could have on the patients with schizophrenia when they visited. His observations of the families varied significantly from those reported by the patients he was seeing in treatment.

During his years at the Menninger Foundation, Bowen undertook a number of observational studies, one of which is described in the paper "A Psychological Formulation of Schizophrenia" (1995). These observations and his wide reading in the natural sciences laid the groundwork for his research at the Family Study Project at NIMH. From the beginning, the clinical work was a basic element in his research both at the Menninger Foundation, later at NIMH, and then at Georgetown University. Observations from psychotherapy with the schizophrenic patients and their families as well as families with lessor symptoms seen on an outpatient basis played a significant role in the development and testing of hypotheses. The original hypothesis in the Family Studies Project was based on the symbiosis between mothers and their adult child with schizophrenia.

> The working hypothesis, formulated from experience with mothers and patients individually, had accurately predicted the way each would relate to the other as individuals. It did not predict, or even consider, a large area of observations that emerged from the living-together situation. The "emotional oneness" between mother and patient was more intense than expected. The oneness was so close that each could accurately know the other's feelings, thoughts, and dreams. In a sense they could "feel for each other," or even "be for each other." . . . There were repeated observations to suggest that the mother-patient oneness extended beyond the mother and patient to involve the father and other family members. (Bowen, 1978 p. 72)

A major shift occurred when the hypothesis was changed from an individual orientation involving mother and patient to a "family unit" hypothesis. Early in the Family Study Project each schizophrenic patient was seen in individual psychotherapy by a psychiatrist and the mothers were seen individually by a social worker. Once the family "oneness" could be observed among the families residing on the unit, the psychotherapy was changed and the family was now seen as the unit of treatment (Bowen, 2013a; Butler, 2013).

All individual psychotherapy on the unit was ceased. Once this shift occurred a different order of observations could be made. In addition to the 24/7 observations of the families on the research unit, the family psychotherapy allowed for more detailed observations of family functioning.

Following the NIMH study, Bowen continued to modify the family psychotherapy. One modification entailed a shift from seeing the whole family unit to meeting with just the central triangle of the parents and their symptomatic son or daughter. A later change was to see the parents only. Bowen found that the inclusion of the symptomatic child in the psychotherapy made it difficult for the parents to shift their focus from their child to themselves and their marital relationship. The focus remained on the family emotional system, but more progress was found to occur when only the two heads of the family were seen. The goal in this process is to assist one or both parents to increase their level of differentiation of self in relation to one another. When one or both parents can make some progress, the functioning of the family unit can be observed to pull up.

Another approach to family therapy developed by Bowen involved seeing just one member of the family. This can be a more difficult approach, especially for a therapist not grounded in the theory and who has not had some success in his or her own family. Family therapy with an individual generally involves seeing the family member most motivated for change. The challenge for a therapist is to discern the subjective reports of a family member about the family from a more objective view of the family. This is accomplished through the use of theory and gaining facts of the individual's multigenerational family. It also requires the therapist to monitor his/her own emotional reactions in the effort to maintain emotional neutrality about that individual's family relationship system.

The approaches of meeting with the marital pair or a motivated adult individual have continued to be central in the psychotherapy or coaching based on Bowen theory. But another important development occurred following an effort Bowen had made with his own family and a subsequent report on this effort he made in a presentation at a national Family Research Conference in 1967. In what he later described as an unexpected development, another approach emerged in assisting individuals to increase their level of differentiation of self. Bowen described the effort he made to differentiate himself in his own family of origin in a chapter in a book of the conference presentations (Framo, 1972). The paper was later reprinted in Bowen's own book in a chapter entitled "On the Differentiation of Self" (Bowen, 1978).

Following the national conference, Bowen wrote that he began describing his efforts with his family with the residents in psychiatry he was teaching at Georgetown University Medical School. Without any encouragement on his part, Bowen discovered that the residents began utilizing the concepts on visits home to their parental families. They would later report on their efforts to Bowen in the teaching sessions. The discovery made by Bowen was that the residents appeared to be doing better clinical work as family therapists than the residents who had been engaged in weekly formal family therapy with their spouses. He also observed over time that the children and spouses of the residents making an effort with their parental families also appeared to be making more progress than the families of those residents seen weekly in family therapy.

This had been an unanticipated result from the teaching sessions and was a complete surprise to Bowen. The residents would briefly consult with Bowen about their efforts with their parental families on home visits and he might respond with a few suggestions, but the time involved was minimal. Over the years at Georgetown, Bowen continued to consult with psychiatric residents and other mental health professionals. The coaching of individuals who principally focused on their families of origin became a common practice. Several years after the original "surprise" Bowen wrote:

> The experience with the psychiatric residents in the teaching sessions in the 1967 to 1969 period came as a startling revelation at a time when I was committed to the notion that the fastest and best change in psychotherapy came from working out the relationship between self and the one most important other person in one's life. Here was an experience that contradicted a central theoretical and therapeutic premise. Here was a group, of some fifteen to twenty trainees who met once a week, in which the primary focus was on the primary triangle with the trainee and his parents. None of the trainees or their spouses were in any kind of "therapy." These conferences had no "therapeutic" objective. . . . These residents, and other trainees in the course, were making as much or more progress at change with their spouses and children than similar residents I was seeing weekly in formal family therapy. (Bowen, 1978 p. 533)

DIFFERENTIATION OF SELF IN ONE'S OWN FAMILY

The above experience led to the development of an approach to "bypass the nuclear family" and focus on one's family of origin and multigenerational families. This approach has been standard in the training of mental health professionals interested in using Bowen theory in their practice ever since. Bowen believed that professionals providing family therapy had a responsibility to make the effort to work on themselves in their own families. It is seen as a central undertaking for those interested in practicing Bowen theory-based family therapy.

Bowen developed a postgraduate program on family systems theory and therapy in the department of psychiatry in 1969. The program continued at the later founded Georgetown University Family Center which later became a free-standing organization and is now known as The Bowen Center for the Study of the Family in Washington, DC. A number of other centers providing training in Bowen theory have also developed around the country and overseas by graduates of the Bowen Center postgraduate program. Central to all the programs is the effort to work at differentiation of self in one's own family of origin.

Bowen theory posits that the family is the primary context for development, and it is in that context that the adaptive capacity and functioning of individuals is shaped. The variation in the maturity an individual attains is equivalent to the level of differentiation of self. It remains fairly stable on reaching young adulthood, though it is potentially modifiable with a sustained and disciplined effort by an individual. The concept of differentiation of self describes the variation among individuals in the degree of maturity they have attained. Bowen used the term "unresolved emotional attachment" to describe the degree of emotional dependence on the parental family that remains for an individual throughout life. Individuals replicate their unresolved emotional attachment with their marital partners and in relation to their children. The effort to increase one's level of differentiation is seen as occurring in the context of the family. It is not a solely intellectual process and requires an engagement with family. Based on the theory and the engagement with family, Bowen developed an approach for an individual to work at defining a self in one's family emotional system.

In order to progress in this process, a person generally has to first come to recognize the level of interdependence in the family, how deeply embedded in it he or she is. Some people recognize this intuitively, based on their experience when visiting their families. It is not uncommon for someone to think fondly of their family and look forward to a visit home, only to run up against old patterns which emerge during the visits. This can involve the discomfort of conflicts or the disappointment of the emotional distance they experience with family members after a day or two. They may find their parents being "parental" to which they respond in a less than mature way. They may blame their parents for not accepting them as an adult, while not recognizing how their own emotional dependence underlies their own reactions and behavior. Or they may find themselves "shutting down" and unable to relate as freely as they would like once they engage with their family, blaming themselves for the emergence of old relationship patterns. Their fond thoughts of family may recede into a looking forward to the more comfortable distance they will experience on ending the visit.

Other people may be unaware of their emotional reactivity to their family. Emotional distance is maintained through superficial contact and accepted as the status quo. In such families the relationships may remain friendly, but little of their more personal thoughts or feelings are expressed. It is difficult to recognize the underlying emotional processes at play. Some may feel lonely in the midst their family, while others feel quite comfortable with the established family patterns. The metaphor of a fish trying to see water captures the difficulty in observing relationship patterns and the emotional process which underlies them. I believe that a theory is required to guide one in the effort to observe self and the family.

Relationship patterns are difficult to change and it can often take an upsetting event or a transitional shift in the family to motivate a person to undertake an effort. I believe that the death of my father, followed a few years later by the approaching birth of my first child, played a significant part in my motivation to initiate some change in myself in a way that might contribute to my functioning and that of the next generation. Given the recognition that I was a part of an ongoing multigenerational family process, I believed that I had some responsibility to the next generation to make an effort to grow up a bit more. All families exhibit an emotional equilibrium maintained by the behaviors and functional position of each member. As mentioned in chapter 8, the unresolved emotional attachment of an individual is managed to a significant degree through emotional cutoff, which is a major obstacle in observing the family. The emotional distance maintained through either geography or intrapsychic distancing allows one to maintain a degree of comfort and to avoid the discomfort inherent in one's unresolved attachment with the parental family. For most, emotional cutoff entails a level of denial about one's own unresolved emotional dependence and so an important step in the effort to increase differentiation of self involves gaining some awareness of one's cutoff and then working toward overcoming it. And since cutoff has allowed one to manage the discomfort related to emotional dependence on the parental family, it also requires developing an awareness of that discomfort and a way to tolerate it in moving toward the family.

Murray Bowen developed a method one can undertake to become knowledgeable about one's family, how one functions in it, how one can increase one's functioning, and contribute to the future generations. The approach is based on Bowen theory, Bowen's experience in his effort to differentiate in his own family, and the observation of individuals making this effort over the years. It is not a short-term process, though intermittent progress can be observed along the way. Although some people can experience a certain level of exuberance when first undertaking the effort, a significant level of resistance within self and in the family can be expected. Given that the family system involves an emotional equilibrium, influencing and being influenced by multiple levels involving biological, psychological, and relationship factors, an effort to change can result in a disturbance in the equilibrium and compensatory responses to change back and reestablish the former equilibrium. The simple effort to be in contact with a family member who has been emotionally distant and cut off from the family may disturb the previous relationship balance and stir up emotional reactions not only in one's self but in other family members.

There is a degree of predictability about families which permits one to make an effort to differentiate in a thoughtful and planned manner. The use of a coach with experience in the effort is advisable and can save one from many of the unproductive attempts one can make in a family. A coach can assist one in pursuing more productive pathways and in avoiding the numerous potential pitfalls along the way. Bowen developed a number of basic principles and methods for making the effort to define a self in one's family of origin. I will list a number of these principles and techniques which can also be found in a chapter in Bowen's book entitled "Toward the Differentiation of Self in One's Family of Origin" (1978) and in Daniel Papero's 1990 book. A discussion of this topic can also be found in two videotaped interviews of Murray Bowen by Michael Kerr in 1980 titled "Defining a Self in One's Family of Origin. Parts 1 and 2." They can be accessed through The Bowen Center for the Study of the Family website, www.thebowencenter.org.

THE FAMILY DIAGRAM AND FAMILY HISTORY

In most forms of psychotherapy, it is the therapeutic relationship which is seen as central in the effort to change. Bowen theory posits that the most basic change involves the effort to increase one's level of differentiation of self, and that this change occurs in relation to one's family. A coach, grounded in Bowen theory, can serve as a resource in the effort, but the responsibility lies with the individual interested in making the effort and the primary relationship in this process is with the family and not the coach.

Basic to the effort to define a self is getting to know one's family. The interest in getting to know one's family may sound odd to some. We grow up in a family and most people stay in some contact with family members throughout their lives. Who would we know better? Developing some objectivity about the family, its members, and one's self, however, is a different matter. One's involvement in family from birth and the automaticity of relationship patterns contribute to the difficulty in gaining some objectivity. Our observational blindness is based on the biases we pick up from others and our early experiences. And, as mentioned, developing the capacity to think systems is key. Family is the principal environment during the course of development and it is evident that that experience shapes our very perceptions of the world, ourselves, and especially of those with whom we have been most involved.

If Bowen theory is accurate, we are born into a functional niche which has been unfolding even prior to our parents' births and their parents' births. We inherit more than our genes and it can be accurate to say that differentiation of self is a multigenerational process (Noone, 2014). As predictable and automatic as this process is, humans have the capacity to learn about and observe the family emotional process at play in their families and the potential to modify their adaptive capacity to some degree. From this perspective, a first step in the effort to increase one's differentiation is to become knowledgeable about the multigenerational families of which we are a part. Bowen theory would posit that the multigenerational family emotional process is alive and well in the present. Gaining knowledge about the larger extended family and the previous generations appears to be necessary in the effort to observe what is right in front of our eyes.

As mentioned, Bowen's own interest in the multigenerational family history grew out of the Family Study Project at NIMH. He wrote,

> Early in family research I began structured studies to trace the transmission of family characteristics from one generation to another. This was part of the effort to define the "the multigenerational transmission process," one of the concepts in the theory. . . . .Thousands of hours went into a microscopic study of a few families, in which I went back as far as 200 or 300 years, and I traced the histories of numerous families back 100 years or more. All families seemed to have the same basic patterns. This work was so time-consuming that I decided it was more sensible to study my own family. (Bowen, 1978 p. 491)

Over a period of ten years, Bowen described gaining knowledge about 24 families of origin in his multigenerational family history, including considerable knowledge of several going back more than 200 years. He was interested in gaining as much factual knowledge as possible about the families and their members from the most adaptive to the least. Bowen came to consider the gathering of knowledge about one's multigenerational family history as vital to the effort to define a self in one's family.

> It is difficult to estimate the direct contribution of family's historical information to the understanding of one's family in the present. I believe the indirect contributions are great enough to warrant the effort by anyone who aspires to become a serious student of the family. In only 150 to 200 years an individual is the descendent of 64 to 128 families of origin, each of which has contributed something to one's self. With all the myths and pretense and emotionally biased reports and opinions, it is difficult to ever really know "self" or to know family members in the present or recent past. As one reconstructs facts of a century or two ago, it is easier to get beyond the myths and to be factual (Bowen, 1978 p. 492).

The details of any multigenerational family history can be enormous, exponentially growing with each of the previous generations. In the study of families on the research unit at NIMH, Bowen developed the use of a family diagram to capture relevant facts about the families. The diagram includes the pertinent facts of a family and how they are related. It also can include some graphics which capture relationship patterns in each nuclear family. A goal in gathering the family history is to obtain a nuclear family history going back as far as possible. An example of a family diagram is illustrated in figure 10.1. There are some slight variations among those using family diagrams and the illustrations here are those which I have used. A manual for developing a family diagram during the coaching process was written by Victoria Harrison (2018), Director, Center for the Study of Natural Systems and the Family. The diagram allows for more than genealogical information. Figures 10.2 and 10.3 illustrate the symbols used in creating a family diagram. A family diagram app has also been developed (https//.www.familydiagram.com) by Patrick Stinson at Alaska Family Systems.

Once sufficient facts are gathered for a family, the diagram can permit one to assess both the nuclear family's emotional patterns as well as patterns occurring from generation to generation. The recording of nodal events, such as births, marriages, deaths, and so on, along with the health, education, and occupations of individuals, can shed some light on relationship patterns and the adaptive capacity of families and their members. The diagram also provides one with a view of what data might be missing. The compilation of a family history, guided by theory, can provide a more objective view of the family and allow one to go beyond some of the more subjective views of some members which

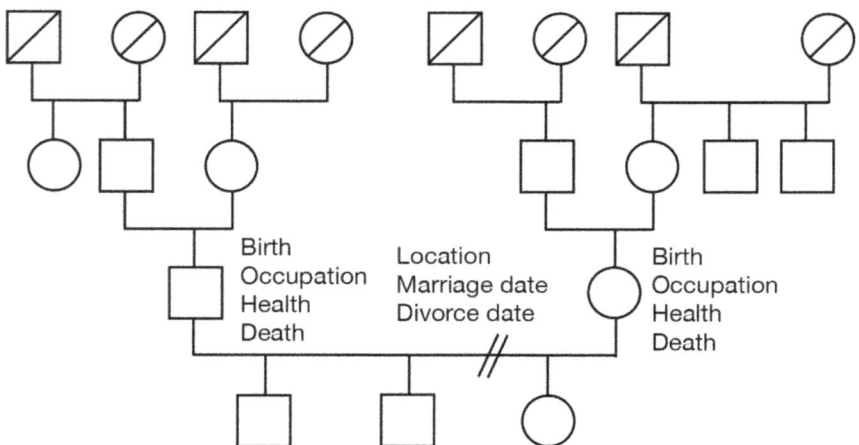

Figure 10.1   A Family Diagram with Relationship and Individual Data. *Source:* Created by the author.

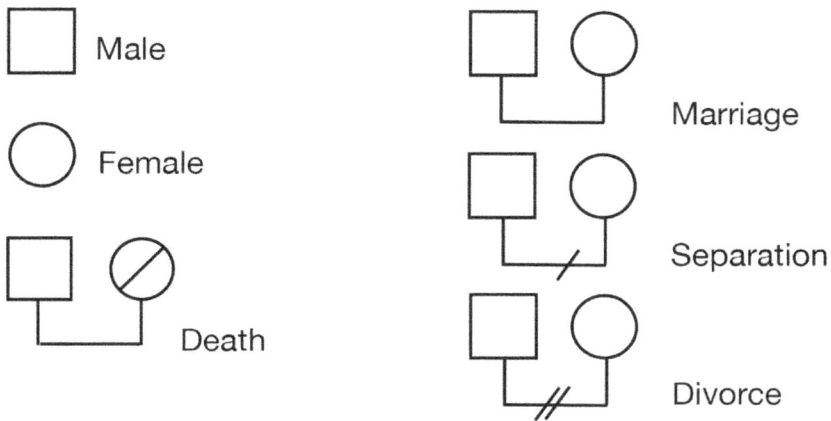

Figure 10.2 Family Diagram Symbols. *Source:* Created by the author.

have been transmitted over one or more generations. As Bowen once described it, a goal is "to take the saints out of heaven and the sinners out of hell."

In addition to obtaining factual knowledge of the family, the family history project also has a process element. The gathering of genealogical information entails being in contact with family members in obtaining information. In a sense it is a technique for coming to know family members and getting their views on other members and events. Obtaining a history has been a useful way of engaging individual family members. It provides a way to have contact with close or distant relatives. A family member, for example, who may have been more cut off from the larger family may be more open to inquiries about family history than he or she would be regarding more personal questions about themselves or others. In the process of interviewing people, a good deal more than facts can be obtained. It can itself be an important process of developing a more personal relationship with individual members of the extended family. A common experience for many in gathering family data and adding it to their family diagram is that patterns, previously unseen, often emerge with the addition of new facts. Knowledge about events and shifts in relationships following the death of a great grandparent, for example, may now add clarity to what had been seen as unrelated events. For most, a new level of respect for the family and its members occurs when they are viewed in the broader context of their lives.

BECOMING A BETTER OBSERVER

An effort to know the family requires developing an ability to become a better observer of the family and one's self. As social creatures we are highly

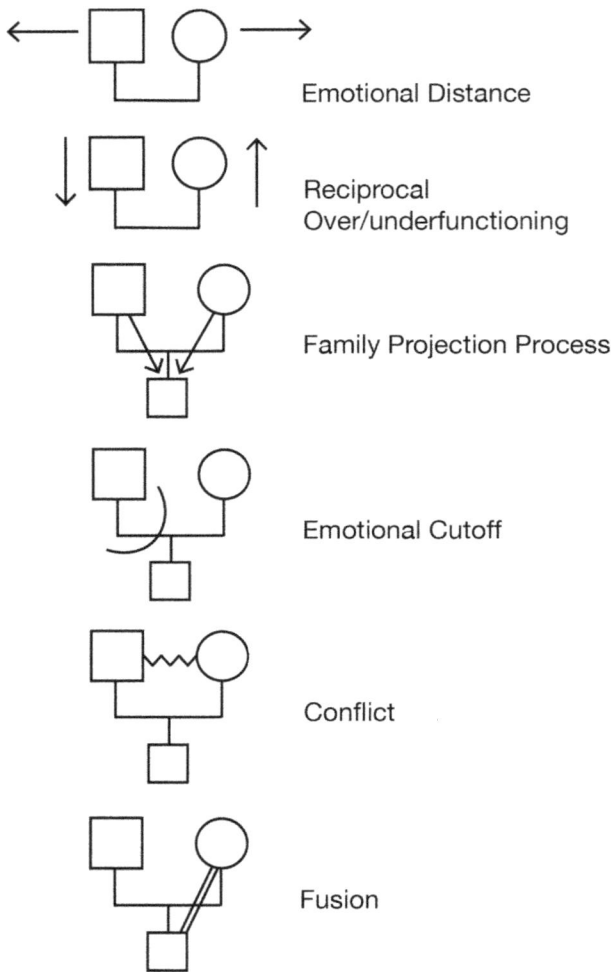

Emotional Distance

Reciprocal
Over/underfunctioning

Family Projection Process

Emotional Cutoff

Conflict

Fusion

Figure 10.3   Emotional Process Symbols. *Source:* Created by the author.

responsive when engaged with others, especially those most important to us and our family. Whether at a family gathering or with an individual family member, our responsiveness to others can make it difficult to observe relationship processes. Becoming a better observer of both self and others in an emotional system is a skill one can learn. It does not mean being distant or aloof, but of increasing one's awareness of what is occurring during interactions. It requires developing a research mindset, a mindset of curiosity. It is not possible to be completely objective in a family setting, but the effort can allow one to get a bit more on the outside of the emotional system. A mindset of curiosity can allow one to be both engaged and observant. The emotional system is in a constant state of flux and its complexity can be a marvel to behold. The effort to become a better observer of the family also influences how one participates in the family. Observing the emotional system requires the activation of higher cortical systems which in itself can have a calming effect.

REGULATING EMOTIONAL REACTIVENESS

A goal of becoming a better observer entails observing one's self and one's emotional reactivity, especially in the context of relationship systems. Can you learn more about how others influence your behavior and your emotional reactions? Are you more comfortable moving toward some and away from others? Are you aware of your own level of tension or anxiety in the group? Do you go quiet or become a chatterbox? The family emotional system includes our own automatic emotional functioning. Basic to the effort of differentiation is the ongoing effort to manage one's emotional reactivity in the relationship system. When one can make progress in observing one's emotional reactivity, it becomes possible to make gains in regulating that reactivity. As with most complex skills, this can require practice over time. If one's natural tendency is to go silent or recede into the background at a family gathering, for example, an effort to engage another can be practiced. Initially such an effort may increase one's anxiety, but over time it is possible to modify the behavior and the anxious feelings.

It is important to note that regulating one's emotional reactivity does not necessarily mean being calm. It may entail making an effort in the family which will increase one's anxiety and then require an effort to contain it. If you have the impression that a family member is uninterested in talking with you, for example, it may initially require managing a feeling of rejection. Any effort to interact in a manner that differs from an automatic pattern generally increases anxiety. It is the avoidance of anxiety that frequently inhibits an effort to become more knowledgeable about the family and develop more personal relationships with family members. Since many patterns are predictable, it can be possible to go "against the current," be aware of how you will react, and not allow the feelings to become an obstacle in undertaking a new behavior. A trainee in a postgraduate program recently gave such an example. He mentioned that a common pattern at family gatherings was that of his older sister criticizing him. His usual response had been to defend himself or counterattack. He went into a family meeting with a plan to respond differently. When his sister predictably criticized him during a family discussion, he was able to inhibit his usual responses and come back with a neutral response. He said in doing this he became tensed but managed to contain his tension. This may sound like a trivial effort, but it is an example of seeing a family pattern, one's part in it, and then not responding automatically.

The effort to define a self in one's family requires that it be undertaken for self. If it represents an effort to change another or attempt to persuade another to accept one's view on an issue, it will not contribute to differentiation. The family emotional system entails relationship patterns which sustain an emotional equilibrium. A successful effort to define a self in the family requires learning about one's part in contributing to the patterns which sustain that equilibrium. Emotional reactivity or stress can quickly override the ability to observe others, but especially that of one's self. For this reason, it is important to work at increasing the capacity to observe one's emotional reactivity and then become more adept at regulating it. Since much of an individual's emotional reactivity operates outside of awareness, it generally requires a conscious effort to learn more about how it is expressed, physiologically and behaviorally. There is no better arena for making this effort than during important family gatherings.

NODAL EVENTS

A general rule of thumb in gaining knowledge of the family and defining a self is the importance of "showing up" for important family events whenever possible. Such events, referred to as "nodal," include all of those gatherings which represent a change or shift in the family. They include funerals, weddings, bar mitzvahs, baptisms, and other transitions in a family's life. In some families this happens as a matter of course. In others it occurs less frequently in the extended family. Often reasons are cited regarding nonattendance at extended family nodal events. "I really don't know them that well and I might just be an intrusion during their time of grief." "The time and travel expense involved in making it to their wedding just don't seem worth it." "I'm too busy at present to be there." There can be valid reasons for not making it to a family nodal event, but often the reasons represent an internal resistance, allowing one to avoid the perceived unpleasant tension of being in contact with segments of the family or of being present during an emotionally charged time. It is interesting to note how pleased people usually are when they override their reluctance and attend a family funeral or wedding occurring in the extended family.

There are a number of reasons for the importance of attending family nodal events. One is that because the events are important to segments of the family, people are often more open with one another and there is a greater potential for developing more of a personal relationship with one or more family members at such times. Another is that during emotionally important family events, relationship patterns may be more evident than at other times. Conflicts, alliances, and cutoffs may be more apparent when families come together. Often one learns about other events previously unknown, such as the birth of a cousin's child, a divorce, or the diagnosis of a serious illness. And probably most important is that of becoming a more active member of the larger family and becoming known to others as an interested family member. Attendance at nodal events can set the stage for being a more responsible family member and being recognized as such by the family. It is in this effort that one gains a clearer view of being a part of a larger family system.

In addition to attendance at family nodal events in the present, the recording of past nodal events on the family diagram plays a vital part in learning about the events that influence the functioning of families and their members. Dates that once seem unrelated a generation or two ago can "light up" family emotional processes which continue into the present. It can become clearer, for example, why one branch of the family has little or no contact with another. The adaptive capacity of individuals and their families in the past can become more obvious in relation to the important events of the time. Such knowledge can contribute to an increasing respect for family members and a greater appreciation that each was "doing the best they could" given the circumstances of their lives. The participation in family nodal events in the present and the recording of those in the past are vital elements on the path to increase one's adaptive capacity or differentiation of self.

PERSON-TO-PERSON RELATIONSHIPS

One of the basic operating principles Bowen presented for anyone motivated to work at defining a self in one's family involved an overall objective of attempting to develop a personal, one-to-one relationship with members of the immediate and extended family. The challenge is simple in description only. As Bowen writes,

> In broad terms, a person to person relationship is one in which two people can relate personally to each other about each other, without talking about others (triangling), and without talking about impersonal "things." Few people can talk personally to anyone for more than a few minutes without increasing anxiety, which results in silences, talking about others, or talking about impersonal things. In its ultimate sense, no one can ever know what a person to person relationship is, since the quality of any relationship can always be improved. On a more practical level, a person to person relationship is between two fairly differentiated people who can communicate directly, with mature respect for each

other, without the complications between people who are less mature. The effort to work toward person to person relationships improves the relationship system in the family and it is a valuable exercise in knowing self. (Bowen, 1978 p. 540)

While the goal of developing a person-to-person relationship with all the members of the extended family may be practically impossible, it provides a direction. The members of all families maintain a certain degree of emotional distance necessary for their personal comfort. The difficulty in making the effort to develop a person-to-person relationship becomes evident once it is made. If, for example, such an effort is made with an uncle, he may quickly pull in his spouse or she may insert herself. A cousin may invite a sibling to a planned visit with just him or her. Addressing a letter to a relative without including their spouse may seem strange and uncomfortable. But, in general, even though there may be a degree of resistance, people come to sense that you are interested in them and in their life. Another advantage of making this effort is in learning more about one's own resistance to engaging in a more personal relationship with a family member. Some relationships are relatively easy, while others stir up an unanticipated level of anxiety. Without knowing it, one can stumble onto a family triangle that had not been activated for years. Or it may be an indicator of an emotional cutoff that had existed in a previous generation. And the effort to develop a person-to-person relationship with extended family members will certainly increase one's awareness of one's own tendency to cutoff.

While a true person-to-person relationship may not be possible with a number of family members, it is possible to develop more open relationships with a good deal of extended and immediate family members. This takes the form of knowing to a greater or lesser extent what is going on in their lives and that they learn more about what is taking place in your life. It can take the form of knowing what is going on in their immediate family, that is, births, illnesses, their views on various topics, and so on. There is a value in having more open relationships with the extended family which can translate into better emotional, relationship, physical, and intellectual functioning. And when one person can do this in the family it automatically opens up the larger family system to a degree.

THE PARENTAL TRIANGLE AND EXPANDING THE LENS

It can be said that each of us is born into a parental triangle. This triangle varies with each sibling. And each child is born into a different relationship configuration. They are born into a different time in a family's life and a different time in the parents' marital relationship. Parents will engage their first child differently than their second. A second child may be born into a more stressful time in the parents' life resulting in a different level of emotional involvement. The factors influencing the variation in each parental triangle are many and each triangle can be said to influence the emotional programming of a child throughout their development. Other triangles can be important in influencing a child's development, but the parental triangle is central for most.

Although a number of factors influence the parental involvement of a child in their marital relationship, it is the level of fusion or undifferentiation in the marital pair which most significantly influences the emotional maturation of a child. While the concept of the family projection process describes the relationship pattern in which one child is selected to be more involved in the parental undifferentiation, every child in the family unit is involved to a greater or lesser degree. Another way of describing this is that while the level of unresolved emotional attachment may be greatest with one child, each sibling arrives at adulthood with some level. The level of parental immaturity can be seen as establishing a baseline of maturity from which the offspring will vary. Michael Kerr (2019) describes this parental triangle in writing:

> The triangle pattern describes how potential anxiety in the marital relationship can shift out of that relationship and into the parents' relationships with the children. Because the mother is usually the primary caretaker for the child, her relationship with the child is usually more intense than the father's. This makes the mother-child relationship the most direct influence on transmitting the parental undifferentiation to the child. The anxiety flows most through that relationship, but that anxiety is not inherent in the mother. It is a product of the context in which she lives. The relationship with her husband is a critically important part of that context. . . . It is not about the mother—it is about the parental triangle and the larger context in which it exists. (p. 36)

From this perspective, an ultimate goal in the effort to define a self involves detriangling from one's parental triangle. At a basic level, the goal is to develop a separate one-to-one relationship with each parent. Most commonly people have more of an up close, emotional relationship (positive or negative) with mother and a more distant one with father. The effort to have a separate relationship with each parent, generally highlights the degree to which one is involved and the difficulty in altering one's functioning in the triangle. Each effort will predictably result in a counter move to restore the relationship balance. An effort to move closer to a more distant father will typically result in a response by mother to maintain the "inside" relationship with her son or daughter, a move which father may even support by distancing or pulling his wife into the process.

Because the parental triangle functions in a predictable manner, it is possible to learn about it and function differently within it. In order to do this, however, one has to be able to observe the triangle. For most, the level of emotional involvement and the automaticity of the triangle make it difficult to observe. It is for this reason that gaining knowledge of the extended family and the multigenerational history become essential steps in observing the close-in parental triangle. The parental triangle also does not exist in a vacuum but is itself embedded in the interlocking triangles of the larger family. In writing about his own effort with his parents, Bowen (1978) describes some of this challenge:

> Time with each parent alone is essential for establishing an individual relationship, but mere private talk with a single parent can accomplish little. One has to be aware that one was "programmed" into the system long ago and it is automatic for both parties to fall back on familiar patterns. An optimal condition for such a relationship is to find a subject of interest to both that does not involve the rest of the family. Each person has his own built-in resistance to working at such a relationship. (p. 502)

He goes on to describe the importance of taking the interlocking triangles into account:

> Up to this point in my family effort, I had incorrectly assumed that I could differentiate a self from my family of origin by differentiating a self from my parents. I believed that if I accomplished this step well I would not have to bother with all the other triangles in which my parents were embedded. The notion about interlocking triangles had been in use almost ten years but I had not integrated this aspect of the theory into the work with my own family (p. 502).

When it is possible to learn more about the parents' families of origin and the grandparents' families, a better vantage point can be gained in observing a parents' relationship with his or her family. Theory also serves as a guide in exploring one's primary triangle. Each parent occupied a functional position in their family of origin. What relationship patterns were at play in their nuclear families? Is it possible to learn more about their unresolved attachment to their parents? What can be learned about the grandparents' families and the positions they occupied? What events might have contributed to the intensity of family triangles in the past? Can you observe the parental triangles of your siblings? As Kerr writes, "Triangles are forever, at least in families. Once the emotional circuitry of a triangle is in place, it usually outlives the people who participate in it" (Kerr & Bowen, 1988 p. 135).

The ability to observe self participating in the parental triangle is gained slowly over time. The detriangling effort, however, requires more than observing. It requires gaining some neutrality about the parents' relationship. All sorts of biases about the parents and their relationship can contribute to how one participates in the triangle. One parent can be viewed as warm, the other as distant or cold. They can be seen as strong/weak, healthy/sick, victim/abuser. How does the functional position of each influence your relationship with them? A significant aspect of detriangling involves coming to see the reciprocity in their relationship.

In addition to gaining some neutrality about the parental relationship, detriangling requires engagement and maintaining that neutrality. Taking sides or going silent is evidence of being triangled. Being engaged, not taking sides, and not distancing are important aspects of the process. The processes involved in most parental triangles are quite subtle and often may not entail conflict or stated differences between the parents. It may involve a comfortable closeness with mother and an equally comfortable distance with father. The emotional process may involve little that is verbal and be principally sustained by nonverbal behavior. An effort to detriangle will disturb that comfort and the effort to define a self in relation to the parents requires an ability to act out of self with each parent as opposed to responding based on the automatic signaling occurring in the relationship. When one family member can make some progress in detriangling, in defining more of a self, the relationships become more open. The family gains a bit more flexibility or adaptive capacity.

The parental triangle involves the level of fusion existing in the parents' marriage and the extent to which one is involved in that fusion. It can be difficult to observe the fusion due to the emotional distance existing in the marital relationship of one's parents. The distance itself is reflective of the fusion. Divorced parents can represent different challenges for individuals seeking to detriangle from their parents. In some families, the emotional intensity may remain high and the effort to develop a relationship with the "outside" parent may stir up a good deal of tension for each member of the triangle. In others, it may be easier to have separate personal relationships when the parents have been divorced, though the effort to do so can often stir what had been a dormant emotional reactivity.

Bowen noted the importance of an experienced coach or guide in the effort to develop an individual relationship with parents:

> Many different kinds of problems are encountered in the effort to develop an individual relationship with each parent. This is where it is desirable to have a "coach" who has already had the experience with his own family. Without such help, one unwittingly makes critical decisions based on emotionality and

can waste months in fruitless dead-ends. A coach who has had experience can at least guide the trainee away from unprofitable trial and error wandering. (Bowen, 1978 pp. 540–541)

Bowen also noted the importance in making an effort to develop a personal relationship with family members to go by oneself on visits.

> It is far better if people go alone to visit their families. A differentiating effort is one that takes place in one self in relation to each other self. It is common for family members to be identified as part of groups and cliques, and for people to relate to the groups rather than to individuals. (Bowen, 1978 p. 541)

The value of visiting as an individual to visit a family member was brought home to me on my very first effort to go by myself to meet with an extended family member. I had just begun the postgraduate program at Georgetown in 1975 and I thought that a good person to start with was a paternal great aunt who was in her early 90s at the time. She was the youngest sister of my grandfather who had emigrated to the United States in 1900. She was the last surviving member of that generation and I wanted to see how much family history I could gain from her. But I also had heeded the suggestion from Dr. Bowen to attempt to develop an individual relationship with as many family members as possible.

I had known this great aunt as a child when we visited her several times a year, but I had not seen her in a number of years. With a good deal of trepidation, I had called her to request a visit and so even though she had expected me, she was quite startled when she opened her door. She relaxed when I said who I was and she responded, "I didn't recognize you without your mother!" The value of visiting family on my own has remained with me and this first visit helped me to overcome my jitters in making such an effort with many other family members over the years.

DETRIANGLING SELF FROM EMOTIONAL SITUATIONS

One of the most profitable efforts with family is to be present during emotionally difficult times. This can take place when a conflict or cut off has occurred in certain segments of the family or during a troubled time such as a death in the extended family. Such occasions can at times permit the opportunity to detriangle self with important others. Bowen writes,

> This is an absolute necessity if differentiation of self is the goal. All the work that goes into personal relationships, as well as into learning more about the

family through observation and into controlling one's own reactiveness, helps both to create a more "open" relationship system and to reactivate the emotional system as it was before one's cutoff from it. Now it is possible to see the triangles in which one grew up, and be different in relation to them. . . . There are many details to this process. One part of the process is achieved merely by being in the midst of the family during an emotional issue, and being more objective and less reactive than the others. The family "knows" this when it happens. (Bowen, 1978 p. 542)

SIBLINGS

For most, the relationship with one's siblings is lifelong. Siblings have also been active participants in the "undifferentiated ego mass" one grew up in. Tense, distant, or conflictual sibling relationships are commonplace and individuals seeking to differentiate a self in their family of origin often focus on these primary relationships. It is also commonplace for two siblings to be in the close inside leg of a triangle with another on the outside.

A guiding principle in the differentiating effort is that it is generally more productive when the effort takes place in relation to one's parents and the previous generations than with one's siblings. When, for example, a father has been especially distant, a triangle between two siblings and their mother may appear primary based on the level of emotional reactivity that is observed. Father's distance, of course, is a significant part of that triangle. Though the reactivity may be more immediately reactive, it generally represents a process the origins of which can be observed in the previous generation or two. Siblings, however, can occupy an important position in the triangle with a parent. The observation of a triangle involving self, a sibling, and a parent, along with the effort to detriangle in this relationship pattern, can play an important part in the process of differentiating a self in relation to one's parents.

A common pattern, for example, can be a triangle consisting of mother, a focused-upon sibling and another sibling (figure 10.4). One sibling (A) may be the focus of maternal anxiety while another (B) might be emotionally involved in the relationship by seeing their sibling as the source of mother's distress. They may then resent their sibling for "causing" mother's distress, being sensitive to her distress, and then responding by attempting to avoid causing mother any further distress. This can result in assuming a functional position of attempting to please mother by operating "under the radar" or being the good or better functioning child. In this example, the focus-upon child is more fused with mother, the other child less fused. One expression of the less-fused child's unresolved emotional attachment with mother may take

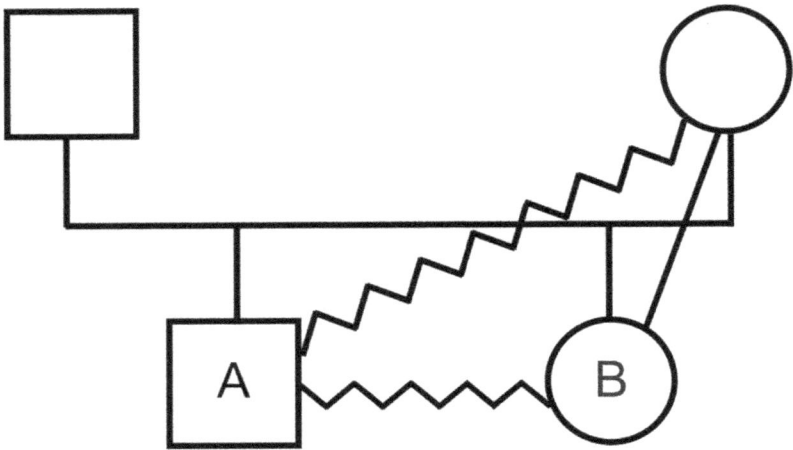

Figure 10.4   Parent–Sibling Triangle. *Source:* Created by the author.

the form of an exaggerated sensitivity to mother's distress, a pattern which continues in his or her other important relationships in adult life.

Detriangling for sibling (B) would involve separating from the emotional intensity of the other mother–child relationship while continuing to relate to both. This would also entail not assuming responsibility for mother's distress regarding the other sibling and gaining some neutrality about the emotional reactivity in their relationship. It does not involve distancing from mother but increasing the capacity to self-regulate while in contact with the distressed mother and the more reactive sibling.

As with the effort to differentiate a self in the parental triangle, success with a parent/sibling triangle is more likely to be achieved when the field of observation is expanded to include the multigenerational family. Given that the triangles in the family of origin are so immediate to our experience and operate so automatically, the study of the multigenerational family can lend a degree of objectivity not possible without it. A central triangle operating in the present generation is seldom unrelated to similar patterns in the previous generations. In the previous example, for example, the mother may have functioned in a similar triangle with a sibling and her mother (figure 10.5). The study of the parent's family of origin and that of previous generations can create a better vantage point for observing the triangle in the present. Knowledge of facts from the previous generation may also contribute to an understanding of the level of reactivity in the current triangle. Overall, however, the triangles at play in previous generations have less emotional intensity for people and so can allow for a more objective view of the process in the present.

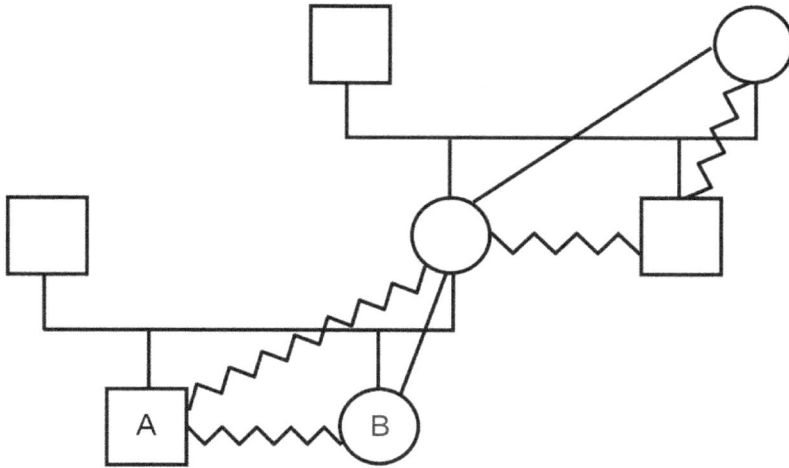

Figure 10.5   Parent–Sibling Triangles over Two Generations. *Source:* Created by the author.

WORK AND OTHER RELATIONSHIP SYSTEMS

All human relationship systems from a Bowen theory perspective are viewed as emotional systems. They vary based on the degree to which the members have ongoing involvement and the extent to which the system and its relationships have importance to the members. For most people, next to the family, their work systems represent a primary emotional system in their lives. Work systems like families vary in their intensity and level of involvement among the members. The intensity and involvement can be felt as positive when, for example, people are engaged in working together for a common goal which they share and are invested in. Each member can see themselves as contributing to a product or mission that is important to them. Being a part of and contributing to an effort larger than oneself is inherently gratifying.

Often a well-functioning "team" is due to the leadership in the organization, but it can also be the mission itself even when the leadership is viewed as lacking or incompetent. Emotional relationship processes exist whether the system is a large corporation involving thousands of employees or smaller systems in which the staff members know one another. Most full-time faculty members of an academic department, for example, will readily agree that it functions as an emotional system. The faculty may be committed to their teaching and deeply invested in contributing to their students' learning and their larger academic field. The stress involved may be seen as acceptable based on a view that their contribution is important to them, their students, and the university. Departments will vary in their esprit de corps, but individual faculty can remain committed to and invested in their work even when a significant degree of disharmony exists in the department.

Another observable example would be that of a restaurant and its staff which function like a well-oiled machine. Staff at all levels are actively engaged and can be observed to interact in a highly integrated manner. The level of cooperation and mutual respect can be observed as each worker contributes to what can be seen as a high-performance art form. There can be a sense of pride in creating a rewarding dining experience for the patrons. The opposite, of course, can also be found at restaurants in which the staff lack a sense of teamwork and carry out their duties with minimal effort. The range in size and complexity of work systems varies, of course, but they are relationship systems and function as emotional systems.

Work systems can be felt by workers as oppressive or negatively stressful and the primary incentive is strictly receiving a paycheck. Employees may feel constrained in their work and the overall energy level is low. Conflicts may exist among and within subunits and the employees look forward to the end of the day every day. There may be a significant level of employee turnover, but the work emotional system continues unchanged. Individual workers may not feel involved, but they will still be influenced by the relationship system of the workplace environment. Emotional patterns exist in all work systems but vary in the employees' functional levels of differentiation, the time and energy required of them, and in the level of chronic anxiety in the organization.

The basic principles involved in the effort to define a self in the family can also apply to the work system, though there are several significant differences between these emotional systems which will influence the effort. A primary one, of course, is related to the position one has in a work system. The head of an organization generally has more capacity to modify their functioning and that of the organization. Others who function in positions of leadership throughout an organization also have more latitude to define a self in their areas of responsibility. For the most part, work systems are not as important to people as their families. Some may put a good deal more life energy into their work and may subjectively feel they are more involved in their career or work system, but the level of emotional dependency of people is typically greater in the family even though they may be unaware of it. There may be times when the level of anxiety or emotional intensity is greater in one's workplace than in their family and require more emotional energy for an individual. And depending on the level of emotional investment, the relationship patterns established in the family of origin are usually replicated in the work system. While more can be gained in the effort to differentiate a self in the family, the effort in a work system can be of great benefit to the individual and generally to the work system as well.

In a brief chapter titled "Toward the Differentiation of Self in Administrative Systems" (Bowen, 1978 pp. 461–465), Bowen described a basic principle he had arrived at. He believed that if an emotional issue arose in his organization, he must be playing a part in it. The basic principle involved clarifying his responsibility in the organization, not assuming responsibility for others, and modifying the part he played in the issue which had emerged. He observed that when he could accomplish this, others would also do the same. Bowen writes,

> The over-all goal in this paper was to indicate that emotional issues in administrative organizations have the same basic patterns as emotional issues in the family, that it is as accurate to think of varying levels of differentiation in work situations as it is in the family, and that the principles toward the differentiation of self in work situations can be as effective as they are in the family. (Bowen, 1978 p. 464)

Organizational charts do not capture the emotional relationship patterns in an organization, but most people are aware of the emotionality that can be involved. During stressful periods in an organization the level of triangling (often taking the form of gossip) and emotional reactivity are running at a higher level. The family adaptive patterns of conflict, distancing, reciprocal over-/under-functioning, and the projection process can be observed. The projection process may involve a focus on one employee who is perceived to be the "problem" by co-workers or administrators. That worker may in fact be performing poorly, but their functioning may decline in response to either over-functioning by others or by the triangling involved in the projection process. How much influence an individual can have on the functioning of the organization will depend to a large degree on their position, but most people can make a gain for themselves and in their work unit when they can work toward differentiating a self in that organization. A process in the family, described by Bowen, can also apply in a work system:

> When any key member of an emotional system can control his own emotional reactiveness and accurately observe the functioning of the system and his part in it, and he can avoid counterattacking when he is provoked, and when he can maintain an active relationship with the other key members without withdrawing or becoming silent, the entire system will change in predictable steps. (Bowen, 1978 p. 436)

The study of the family which resulted in the development of Bowen theory also entailed the effort to develop a form of psychotherapy based on the theory. The forms of psychotherapy developed by Bowen evolved as the theory developed. Whole families, the parental couple with the symptomatic child, the marital couple alone, and individuals alone, all represented forms of family psychotherapy. Based on theory, the focus of the therapy was on the family unit and its multigenerational context. A focus on the families of origin increased over time. The discovery by Bowen that "coaching" individuals about their families of origin could be as effective, or even more so, than formal psychotherapy, became the principal mode involved in the training of mental health professionals.

Conclusion

Murray Bowen developed an original theory, moving from a view in which the individual is the focus of study to the family. The theory moved from viewing the human as unique and different from other forms of life, to one which places Homo sapiens as a species among species and a product of its evolutionary heritage. As a systems theory, it incorporates underlying interdependent elements involved in human functioning, from the family and broader relationship systems to the biological substrates of physiology. The family is seen as an adaptive system shaping the development and functioning of its members and an intricate part of its extended and multigenerational families. Individual variation in adaptiveness (differentiation of self) is placed along a continuum related to the extent to which higher cortical systems (defined as the intellectual system) can be utilized in guiding behavior. At one end of the continuum are individuals whose behavior is principally other-regulated in the social environment. At the other end are individuals who have the capacity to regulate their behavior and determine a direction in their life course. The differentiation or maturation of the intellectual system is posited to be a developmental process, shaped largely by the family emotional system. On reaching adulthood, the differentiation of a self in the family is viewed as a relatively stable process. It represents the adaptive capacity of individuals which can be observed in their health, behavior, and overall relationship functioning. Differentiation of self is influential in mate selection and establishes a baseline of maturity from which the next generation will vary.

Bowen theory is a relatively new theory, first published in 1966. It was developed and primarily utilized in the field of mental health. Though I believe that knowledge developing in the natural sciences has been supportive of the theory, the theory remains largely unknown outside of the mental health field. Bowen believed that the acceptance of the theory would not occur for perhaps a hundred years or more. Despite the length of time it has taken to accept the human as a product of evolution and despite the apparent difficulty required in thinking systems, there has been significant progress in that direction in recent decades. Systems thinking has entered mainstream biology and as microbiologist James Shapiro (2011) writes,

> The science of the 21st Century deals with the interactions between the multiple components of complex systems, ranging from aggregates of elementary particles (each of which has its own multivalent set of properties) to the behavior of the largest structures in the cosmos. This kind of science is fundamentally different from earlier periods, when the goal was to understand the unique property of each atomistic unit and then try to derive the behavior of large systems from a small set of interaction rules plus the character of their component parts. Today, a major focus in scientific inquiry is to understand how systems change over time, whether they are atoms, molecules, organisms, ecosystems, climates, galaxies, black holes, or universes. (p. 145)

The complexity of living systems requires that investigators take into account the reciprocal processes occurring at all levels of life. But the inclusion of family as a natural system remains largely excluded as an area of investigation in most disciplines. It is remarkable, for example, that an emerging field such as social neuroscience, which is based on the awareness of the extent to which social processes influence brain development and functioning, does not at this point in time consider the family as a distinct biopsychosocial system central to development. In discussing the multiple levels of influence on the brain from genes to societal processes, the family is largely unmentioned in social neuroscience texts (Cacioppo et al., 2002; Cacioppo, Visser, & Pickett, 2006; Harmon-Jones & Winkielman, 2007). And while advocates of multi-level selection in evolutionary biology advance the view that groups can be units of selection, the family as a unit is not differentiated from other groups (Wilson, 2019). Evolutionary psychologists may consider the importance of family in human evolution (Salmon & Shackelford, 2007), but families are for the most part viewed as collections of individuals rather than biological, self-regulating wholes.

If Bowen theory is accurate, and it is certainly not yet proven to be, the lack of the inclusion of the family as a unit among investigators in the life sciences is an interesting question. Can it be that the deep interdependence of individuals in the family unit and the degree to which behavior is regulated by the family makes it difficult to observe? It took more than a century for Darwin's theory that the human was an evolved form of life to be widely accepted. Family relationship systems are even more immediate to our experience and so does the metaphor that "seeing" the family system is similar to "a fish seeing water" hold? My own view is that science, and especially neuroscience, will move in the direction of recognizing the part family plays in human behavior. It is not long ago that the mention of evolution was uncommon in the neuroscience literature. Now it is widespread. The study of the brain necessarily led to the importance of its evolution in order to fully understand its structure and functions. The growing knowledge of the influence of the social environment on brain development and functioning will, I think, similarly lead to the study of the interplay between the family and the brain, in their development, functioning, and evolution.

As a relatively new theory of human behavior, it has not yet been widely tested or scrutinized in the larger world of science. Much about the theory remains to be fully and rigorously explored. Does the theory apply to the entire human population or is it principally based on the observations of families from Western cultures? Does it describe a process more basic than culture? Is the multigenerational family emotional process accurately described? Is the theory's view of mate selection accurate? Will Bowen theory provide a basis for the integration of knowledge emerging in the fields of genetics, epigenetics, and the broader biological disciplines? Will knowledge of psychological and social processes support, modify, or reject the theory?

One of the tests of an important theory is the degree to which it is productive in furthering research and knowledge. Over the past sixty years, countless individuals would give testimony to the value of the theory in gaining knowledge of their families and making headway in enhancing their adaptive capacity. This support, however, does not entail the rigorous testing the theory requires. Knowledge developing in the sciences lends a different kind of support. To date such knowledge has largely contributed to the theory. Much remains to be learned about human behavior and whether Bowen's systems theory of the family plays an important part in that process will be determined in the future.

Our species emerged relatively recently. Part of the tissue of life wrapped around our blue planet, Homo sapiens has come to dominate the biosphere like no other species. For the most part the human has been quite proud of its accomplishments. We have encircled the globe, explored space and the seas, built cities, and elaborate transportation and communication systems. It is reasonable to assume that within reach can be the end to hunger and poverty for our population of billions. With the exception of horrific wars and the exploitation of some populations by others, the extent to which humans have learned to live together and cooperate in densely populated cities is quite amazing. What other primate could quietly tolerate being tightly bunched together with 300 fellow primates on flights of many hours and great distances? Human ingenuity is an astounding phenomenon and as

E. O. Wilson (2012) has remarked, the human has the potential to create a paradise on earth.

We also have a glass half-empty scenario in which our expansionary appetite has come to be so ecologically dominant that we threaten the survival of our own species and many others. Our primate selves may become aware of the imbalance and destruction to life we are creating in the biosphere, but does the human have the ability to limit our growth and avoid our extinction? Does our species have the adaptive capacity to survive our own dominance? What will it require to develop the ability to regulate ourselves in order to live in harmony with the rest of life on which our survival depends? Life does not depend on the human, evidenced by the extreme conditions in which it has been found to exist. Even if we extinct ourselves and a vast number of other species, it is quite clear that life will persist with or without us. Significant changes in climate have been found to underlie the great mass extinctions over the course of evolution. Whether the human manages to avoid contributing to its own extinction is certainly the most important issue our species faces in the present and future.

Our elaborate brains have allowed us to adapt to wide variations in climate. To a great extent we have been able to adapt to our expanding population and at times have been able to get beyond the ravages and accompanying hatreds we have inflicted on each other. But while natural selection has resulted in a remarkable capacity to adapt, Homo sapiens continues to grow and consume in a manner which may lead to its extinction.

While creative technological solutions to address many of the environmental challenges we are faced with will be required, the ability to regulate the human reflexive, instinctual tendencies will also be required. The higher cortical systems of the human likely evolved to enhance the adaptive capacity of individuals in navigating in complex social environments. These same neural systems, however, are vulnerable to be overridden during heightened stress by our earlier evolved threat response systems. As Jaak Panksepp (1998) writes,

> Our higher brain areas are not immune to the subcortical influences we share with other creatures. Of course, the interchange between cognitive and emotional processes is one of reciprocal control, but the flow of traffic remains balanced only in nonstressful circumstances. In emotional turmoil, the upward influences of subcortical emotional circuits on the higher reaches of the brain are stronger than the top down controls. (p. 301)

There are countless examples of humanitarian responses following natural disasters. The human has demonstrated the capacity to function in a highly cooperative fashion and to contribute to the common good. Altruistic responses to unrelated strangers and distant populations have also been a part of the human experience. At the same time, negative reactions to distressed migrant populations have occurred when they are seen as encroaching on our land or well-being. We have inherited not only our recently evolved neocortices but the rest of our evolutionary heritage as well. Despite widespread denial, we remain instinctive, biological creatures vulnerable to responding automatically when threatened. How will populations respond to the widespread disruptions to basic needs such as food and water, to massive migrations, and other environmental crises when they are close to home?

There is, of course, a growing awareness of the impact human growth is having and the risk to our species' survival. In discussing the human's potential for choice, neuroscientist Joaquin Fuster points out that the more recently evolved prefrontal cortex has not only enhanced the human's ability to learn from experience, assess, and adapt to the present but to pre-adapt as well. He writes,

> It is virtually impossible to discuss the cerebral foundation of liberty without dealing with the evolution of the brain. The reason is simple: The capacity of mammalian organisms to modify their environment by choice and to adapt to it by chosen means has grown enormously with the evolutionary growth of certain parts of their brain, the cerebral cortex in particular. Most relevant to our present discourse is the cortex of the frontal lobes. It is indeed a remarkable fact with a touch of cosmic irony that the science of evolutionary neurobiology, which can only "postdict" but not predict, has unveiled in the prefrontal cortex of man the seed of his future, the capacity to predict and to turn prediction into action that will impact on that future and on that of human society. (Fuster, 2013 p. 28)

This capacity allows us to see what the current trajectory will be bringing us if we fail to adapt.

To those unfamiliar with Bowen theory, differentiation of self is often misconstrued as a concept referring only to the individual. It does describe variation among individuals with regards to their basic adaptive capacity, in their ability to regulate the more automatic emotional reactions when it is important to do so. Differentiation of self, however, is also a relationship concept entailing the basic interdependence at play in the family. An individual's level of differentiation is a product of the family relationship system in which it develops and is related to the functioning of the other members of the family and the family unit as a whole. At higher levels of differentiation, the concept refers to individuals who are aware of their relationship interdependence and who demonstrate a keen sense of their responsibility to the family and their fellow citizens. While much will be required of the human population if it is to successfully adapt to the climate changes we have created, knowledge of factors contributing to the development of our adaptive capacity will be important (Harrison, in press). An understanding of the extent to which our emotional system regulates our behavior as well as the potential to increase our capacity to self-regulate will play a part in thoughtfully "pre-adapting" to the major challenges ahead. The best minds of our species will be required to address climate change and develop the range of technological solutions necessary to limit the environmental damage occurring during this Anthropocene era. It will require the very best of human thinking, a level of systems thinking that the human seems capable of. The coming crises will also necessitate taking into account our instinctual, biological selves. The role of the family in shaping our adaptive capacity may be an important element. As Papero et al. (2018) write,

> Knowledge of the principles of functioning of the family emotional system contributes options for the human to chart a course through increasing chronic anxiety arising from increasingly threatened and threatening natural systems. It provides principles of functioning directed toward management of self in relationship to others and using knowledge of emotional systems to guide behavior for the common good.

> . . . The challenge is to shift out of automatic emotionally reactive behavior patterns in spite of the chronic anxiety fueling them, towards thinking and actions based on responsible principles for the long term. This is also what we mean by systems thinking and what we believe is the potential of systems thinking for the human condition. (p. 28)

It remains questionable whether our species will "rise to the occasion" and effect the necessary changes that will be required to put the brakes on our expansionary and acquisitional nature and adapt to the climate crisis we and our descendants are faced with. Our elaborate brains and remarkable capacity to cooperate will be required to the fullest. The adaptive capacity of the human is being tested as never before. Science will play a vital part, but it will require more than the science involved in technological advances. A science of human behavior and the capacity to regulate the automatic emotional system will also play a part. Bowen theory and knowledge of the family in shaping adaptive capacity can play a vital role.

References

Adolphs, R. & Anderson, D. J. (2018). *The neuroscience of emotion: A new synthesis.* Princeton, NJ: Princeton University Press.

Alexander, R. D. (1990). *How did humans evolve?* (Special publication #1). Ann Arbor: University of Michigan, Museum of Zoology.

Allman, J. (1999). *Evolving brains.* New York: Scientific American Library.

Anacker, C., O'Donnell, K. J., & Meaney, M. J. (2014). Early life adversity and the epigenetic programming of hypothalamic-pituitary- adrenal function. *Dialogues in Clinical Neuroscience,* 16: 321–333.

Arnsten, A. F. T. (2009). Stress signaling pathways that impair prefrontal cortex structure and function." *Nature Reviews Neuroscience,* 10: 410–422.

Arnsten, A. F. T., Wang, M. J., & Paspalas. C. D. (2012). Neuromodulation of thought: Flexibilies and vulnerabilities in prefrontal cortical network synapses. *Neuron,* 76: 223–239.

Barrett, J. & Fleming, A. S. (2011). Annual research review: All mothers are not equal: Neural and psychological perspectives on mothering and the importance of individual differences. *Journal of Child Psychology and Psychiatry,* 52: 368–397.

Barrett, L. F. (2017). *How emotions are made: The secret life of the brain.* Boston: Houghton Mifflin Harcourt.

Ben-Jacob, E., Shapira, Y., & Tauber, A. I. (2011). Smart bacteria. In A. Asikainen & W. E. Krumbein (Eds.), *Chimeras and consciousness: evolution of the sensory self.* Cambridge, MA: The MIT Press.

Bentall, R. P. (2004). *Madness explained: Psychosis and human nature.* New York: Penguin Books.

Bentall, R. P. (2009). *Doctoring the mind.* New York: New York University Press.

Bonanno, G. A. (2004). Loss, trauma, and human resilience: Have we underestimated the human capacity to thrive after extremely aversive events? *American Psychologist,* 59: 20–28.

Bowen, M. (1960). A family concept of schizophrenia. In D. Jackson (Ed.), *The etiology of schizophrenia.* New York: Basic Books, Inc.

Bowen, M. (1966). The use of family theory in clinical practice. *Comprehensive Psychiatry*, 7: 345–374.

Bowen, M. (1978). *Family therapy in clinical practice*. New York: Jason Aronson.

Bowen, M. (1988). An odyssey toward science. In M. E. Kerr & M. Bowen (Eds.), *Family evaluation: The role of the family as an emotional unit that governs individual behavior and development*. New York: W. W. Norton & Company.

Bowen, M. (1995). A psychological formulation of schizophrenia. *Family Systems*, 2:1, 17–47.

Bowen, M. (2013a). *The origins of family psychotherapy: The NIMH Family Study Project*. J. Butler (Ed.). Lanham, MD: Jason Aronson.

Bowen, M. (2013b). Subjectivity, Homo sapiens, and science. *Family Systems*, 9:2, 101–106.

Bowen, M. (2017). A systems view of the aging process. *Family Systems*, 13:1, 47–61.

Bowen, M. (2021). The integration of knowledge. *Family Systems*, 15: 149–155.

Bowen, M. & Kerr, M. E. (1980). Defining a self in one's family of origin. Part 1. Bowen-Kerr videotaped interview series. Produced by The Bowen Center for the Study of the Family. Washington, DC.

Bowen, M. & Kerr, M. E. (1980). Defining a self in one's family of origin. Part 2. Bowen-Kerr videotaped interview series. Produced by The Bowen Center for the Study of the Family. Washington, DC.

Boyce, W. T. & Ellis, B. J. (2005). Biological sensitivity to context: I. An evolutionary – developmental theory of the origins and functions of stress reactivity. *Development and Psychopathology*, 17: 271–301.

Boyce, W. T. & Kobor, M. S. (2015). Development and the epigenome: The 'synapse' of gene-environment interplay. *Developmental Science*, 18: 1–23.

Branchi, I., Curley, J. P., D'Andrea, I., Cirulli, E., Champagne, F. A., & Alleva, E. (2013). Early interactions with mother and peers independently build adult social skills and shape BDNF and oxytocin receptor brain levels. *Psychoneuroendocrinology*, 38: 522–532.

Buchanan, T. W., Bagley, S. L., Stansfield, R. B., & Preston, S. D. (2012). The empathetic, physiological resonance of stress. *Social Neuroscience*, 7: 191–201.

Burkart, J. M., Hrdy, S. B., & Van Schaik, C. P. (2009). Cooperative breeding and human cognitive evolution. *Evolutionary Anthropology*, 18: 175–186.

Burkart, J. M. & Van Shaik, C. P. (2010). "Cognitive consequences of cooperative breeding in primates?" *Animal Cognition*, 13: 1–19.

Burkart, J. M., Allon, O., Amici, F., Fichtel, C., Finkenworth, C., Heschl, A., Huber, J., Isler, K., Kosonen, Z. K., Martins, E., Meulman, E. J., Richiger, R., Rueth, K., Spillmann, B., Wiesendanger, S., & van Schaik, C. P. (2014). The evolutionary origin of human hyper-cooperation. *Nature Communications*, DOI: 10.1038/ncomms5747.

Butler, E. A. & Randall, A. K. (2013). Emotional coregulation in close relationships. *Emotion*, 5: 202–210.

Butler, J. F. (2013). Family psychotherapy: The first evolutionary stage during the NIMH Family Study Project. *Family Systems*, 10: 29–42.

Butler, J. F. (2015). The family as an emotional unit concept: Origins and early history. In R. Noone & D. Papero (Eds.), *The family emotional system: An integrative concept for theory, science, and practice.* New York: Lexington Books.

Cacioppo, J. T., Berston, G. G., Adolphs, R., Carter, C. S., Davidson, R. J., McClintock, M. K., McEwen, B. S., Meaney, M. J., Schacter, D. L., Sternberg, E. M., Suomi, S. S., & Taylor, S. E. (2002). *Foundations in social neuroscience.* Cambridge, MA: The MIT Press.

Cacioppo, J. T., Visser, P. S., & Pickett, C. L. (2006). *Social neuroscience: People thinking about people.* Cambridge, MA: The MIT Press.

Cacioppo, J. T. & Patrick, W. (2008). *Loneliness: Human nature and the need for social connection.* New York: W. W. Norton & Company.

Carter, C. S. (2005). Biological perspectives in social attachment and bonding. In C. Carter, L. Ahnert, K. Grossman, S. Hrdy, M. Lamb, S. Porges, & N. Sachser (Eds.), *Attachment and bonding: A new synthesis.* Cambridge, MA: The MIT Press, pp. 85–100.

Champagne, F. A. (2008). Epigenetic mechanisms and the transgenerational effects of maternal care. *Frontiers in Neuroendocrinology, 29*: 386–397.

Champagne, F. A. (2011). Maternal imprints and the origins of variation. *Hormones and Behavior, 60*: 4–11.

Champagne, F. A. & Curley, J. P. (2015). Epigenetic effects of parental care within and across generations. In R. Noone & D. Papero (Eds.), *The family emotional system: An integrative concept for theory, science, and practice.* New York: Lexington Books.

Cole, S. W. (2013). Social regulation of human gene expression: Mechanisms and implications for public health. *American Journal of Public Health, 103*: 584–592.

Conley, D. (2004). *The pecking order: Which siblings succeed and why.* New York: Pantheon Books.

Crews, D. & Noone, R. J. (2015). Early context-dependent epigenetic modifications and the shaping of brain and behavior. In R. Noone & D. Papero (Eds.), *The family emotional system: An integrative concept for theory, science, and practice.* New York: Lexington Books.

Curley, J. P. & Keverne, E. B. (2005). Genes, brains and mammalian social bonds. *TRENDS in Ecology and Evolution. 20*: 561–567.

Curley, J. P. & Champagne, F. A. (2016). Influence of maternal care on the developing brain: Mechanisms, temporal dynamics and sensitive periods. *Frontiers in Neuroendocrinology, 40*: 52–66.

Damasio, A. (1999). *The feeling of what happens: Body and emotion in the making of consciousness.* New York: Harcourt Brace & Company.

Damasio, A. (2010). *Self comes to mind: Constructing the conscious brain.* New York: Pantheon Books.

Damasio, A. (2018). *The strange order of things: Life, feeling, and the making of cultures.* New York: Pantheon Books.

Dettmer, A. M. & Suomi, S. J. (2014). Nonhuman primate models of neuropsychiatric disorders: Influences of early rearing, genetics, and epigenetics. *Institute for Animal Laboratory Research Journal, 55*: 361–370.

Dilalla, L. F., Kagan, J., & Reznick, J. S. (1994). Genetic etiology of behavioral inhibition among 2-year-old children. *Infant Behavior and Development.* 17: 405–412.

Donley, M. G. (2016). Bonding and babies: The evolution of biparental care and the primary triangle. *Family Systems,* 12: 9–28.

Dunbar, R. I. (1998). The social brain hypothesis. *Evolutionary Anthropology,*6: 178–190.

Dunbar, R. I. (2002). The social brain hypothesis. In J. Cacioppo et al. (Eds.), *Foundations in social neuroscience.* Cambridge, MA: The MIT Press, pp. 69–87.

Dunbar, R. I. (2016). *Human evolution: Our brains and behavior.* New York: Oxford University Press.

Edelman, G. M. (2006). *Second nature: Brain science and human knowledge.* New Haven, CT: Yale University Press.

Eisenberger, N. I. (2011). The pain of social disconnection: Examining the shared neural underpinnings of physical and social pain. *Nature Reviews Neuroscience,* doi: 10.1038/nrn3231.

Eisenberger, N. I. & Cole, S. W. (2012). Social neuroscience and health: Neurophysiological mechanisms linking social ties with physical health. *Nature Neuroscience.* 15: 669–674.

Ellis, B. J., Boyce, W. T., Belsky, J., Bakermans-Kranenburg, M. J., & Van Ijzendoorn, M. H. (2011). Differential susceptibility to the environment: An evolutionary-neurodevelopmental theory. *Development and Psychopathology,* 23: 7–28.

Elston, G. N. (2003). Cortex, cognition and the cell: New Insights into the pyramidal neuron prefrontal function. *Cerebral Cortex,* 13: 1124–1138.

Essex, M. J., Klein, M. H., Cho, E., & Kalin, N. H. (2002). Maternal stress beginning in infancy may sensitize children to later stress exposure: Effects on cortisol and behavior. *Biological Psychiatry,*52: 776–784.

Fleming, A. S. (2005). Plasticity of innate behavior: Experiences throughout life affect maternal behavior and its neurobiology. In C. Carter, L. Ahnert, K. Grossman, S. Hrdy, M. Lamb, S. Porges, & N. Sachser (Eds.), *Attachment and bonding: A new synthesis.* Cambridge, MA: The MIT Press, pp. 137–168.

Flinn, M. V. (2005). Culture and developmental plasticity. In K. MacDonald & R. Burgess (Eds.), *Evolutionary perspectives on child development.* Thousand Oaks, CA: Sage, pp. 73–98.

Flinn, M. V. (2006). Evolution and ontogeny of stress response to social challenges in the human child. *Developmental Review,* 26: 138–174.

Flinn, M. V. & England, B. G. (1998). Social economics of childhood glucocorticoid stress response and health. *American Journal of Physical Anthropology,* 102: 33–53.

Flinn, M. V., Ward, C. V., and Noone, R. J. (2005). Hormones and the human family. In D. Buss (Ed.), *Handbook of Evolutionary Psychology.* New York: Wiley, pp. 552–580.

Flinn, M. V., Geary, D. C., & Ward, C. V. (2005). Ecological dominance, social competition, and coalitionary arms races: Why humans evolved exceptional intelligence. *Evolution and Human Behavior,* 26: 10–46.

Flinn, M. V. & Alexander, R. (2007). Runaway social selection in human evolution. In S. Gangestad & J. Simpson (Eds.), *The evolution of mind: Fundamental questions and controversies*. New York: Guilford Press, pp. 249–255.

Flinn, M. V., Quinlan, R. J., Coe, K., & Ward, C. V. (2007). Evolution of the human family: Cooperative males, long social childhoods, smart mothers, and extended kin networks. In C. A. Salmon and T. K. Shackelford (Eds.), *Family relationships: An evolutionary perspective*. New York: Oxford University Press, pp. 16–38.

Flinn, M. V., Ponzi, D., Nepomnaschy, P., & Noone, R. J. (2012). Ontogeny of stress reactivity: Phenotypic flexibility, trade-offs, and pathology. In G. Laviola & S. Macri (Eds.), *Adaptive and Maladaptive Aspects of Developmental Stress*. Berlin: Springer Press.

Fox, S. E., Levitt, P., & Nelson, C. A. (2010). How the timing and quality of early experiences influence the development of brain architecture. *Child Development*, 81: 28–40.

Framo, J. (1972). *Family Interaction: A dialogue between family researchers and family therapists*. New York: Springer Publishing.

Francis, D., Diorio, J., Lio, D., & Meaney, M. J. (1999). Nongenomic transmission across generations of maternal behavior and stress responses in the rat. *Science*, 286: 1155–1158.

Frost, R. (2020). Operationalizing the concept of differentiation of self for family research. In M. Keller & R. Noone (Eds.), *Handbook of Bowen family systems theory and research methods*. New York: Routledge Press, pp. 138–156.

Fuster, J. M. (2002). Frontal lobe and cognitive development. *Journal of Neurocytology*, 31: 373–385.

Fuster, J. M. (2013). *The neuroscience of freedom and creativity*. New York: Cambridge University Press.

Galloway, D. (2020). How emotions are made: Implications for Bowen theory. *Family Systems*, 14: 129–155.

Gazzaniga, M. S. (1992). *Nature's mind: The biological roots of thinking, emotions, sexuality, language, and intelligence*. New York: Basic Books.

Gianaros, P. J., Jennings, J. R., Sheu, L. K., Greer, P. J., Kuller, L. H., & Matthews, K. A. (2007). Prospective reports of chronic life stress predict decreased grey matter volume in the hippocampus. *Neuroimage*, 35: 795–803.

Gilbert, S. F., Sapp, J., & Tauber, A. I. (2012). A symbiotic view of life: We have never been individuals. *The Quarterly Review of Biology*, 87: 325–341.

Gilligan, M., Suitor, J. J., & Pillemer, K. (2015). Estrangement between mothers and adult children: The role of norms and values. *Journal of Marriage and Family*, 77: 908–920.

Gordon, D. M. (2010). *Ant encounters: Interaction networks and colony behavior*. Princeton, NJ: Princeton University Press.

Guerin, P. (1976). *Family therapy: Theory and practice*. New York: Gardner Press.

Gunnar, M. R. 2005. Attachment and stress in early development: Does attachment add to the potency of social regulators of infant stress?" In C. Carter, L. Ahnert, K. Grossman, S. Hrdy, M., Lamb, S. Porges, & N. Sachser (Eds.), *Attachment and Bonding: A New Synthesis*. Cambridge, MA: The MIT Press, pp. 245–255.

Harari, Y. N. (2015). *Sapiens: A brief history of humankind.* New York: HarperCollins.

Harmon-Jones, E. & Winkielman, P. (2007). *Social neuroscience: Integrating biological and psychological explanations of social behavior.* New York: The Guilford Press.

Hrdy, S. B. (1999). *Mother nature.* New York: Pantheon Books.

Harrison, V. (2018). *The family diagram and family research: An illustrated guide to tools for working on differentiation of self in one's family.* Houston, TX: Center for the Study of Natural Systems and the Family.

Harrison, V. (2020). Bowen theory in the study of physiology and family systems. In M. Keller & R. Noone (Eds.), *Handbook of Bowen family systems theory and research methods.* New York: Routledge Press, pp. 138–156.

Harrison, V. (in press). Understanding and managing the impact of climate changes on anxiety: Bowen theory and an evolutionary perspective. *Family Systems.*

Heldstab, S. A., Isler, K., Burkart, J. M., & van Shaik, C. P. (2019). Allomaternal care, brains and fertility in mammals: Who cares matters. *Behavioral Ecology and Sociobiology,* 73: 71. https://doi.org/10.1007/s00265-019-2684-x

Henrich, J. (2020). *The weirdest people in the world: How the West became psychologically peculiar and particularly prosperous.* New York: Farrar, Straus and Giroux.

Hill, K. & Boyd, R. (2021). Behavioral convergence in humans and animals. *Science,* 371: 235–236.

Jones, A. (2014). Epigenetics, social genomics, and Bowen theory. *Family Systems,* 10: 105–127.

Kahneman, D. (2011). *Thinking, fast and slow.* New York: Farrar, Straus and Giroux.

Kandel, E. R. (2006). *In search of memory: The emergence of a new science of mind.* New York: W. W. Norton.

Kerr, M. E. (1992). Physical illness and the family emotional system: Psoriasis as a model. *Behavioral Medicine,* 18: 101–113.

Kerr, M. E. (2019). *Bowen theory's secrets: Revealing the hidden life of families.* New York: W. W. Norton.

Kerr, M. E. (2020). Foreward. In M. Keller & R. Noone (Eds.), *Handbook of Bowen family systems theory and research methods.* New York: Routledge Press, pp. xiv–xx.

Kerr, M. E. & Bowen, M. (1988). *Family evaluation: An approach based on Bowen theory.* New York: W.W. Norton.

Klever, P. (2009). The primary triangle and variation in nuclear family functioning. *Contemporary Family Therapy,* 31: 140–159.

Klever, P. (2015). Multigenerational relationships and nuclear family functioning. *The American Journal of Family Therapy,* 43: 339–351.

Klever, P. (2021). Divergent spouse functioning. *Family Systems,* 15: 103–129.

Kuhn, T. S. (2012). *The structure of scientific revolutions.* Fiftieth Anniversary Edition. Chicago: The University of Chicago Press.

Langsley, D. G., Pittman, F. S., Machotka, P., & Flomenhaft, K. (1968a). Family crisis therapy: Results and implications. *Family Process,* 7(2), 145–158.

Langsley, D. G. & Kaplan, D. M. (1968b). *Treatment of families in crisis*. New York, NY: Grune and Stratton.

Lassiter, L. (2020). Human stress genomics and Bowen theory: Potential for future research. In M. Keller & R. Noone (Eds.), *Handbook of Bowen family systems theory and research methods*. New York: Routledge Press, pp. 120–137.

LeDoux, J. (2002). *Synaptic self: How our brains become who we are*. New York: Viking.

LeDoux, J. (2015). *Anxious: Using the brain to understand and treat fear and anxiety*. New York: Viking.

LeDoux, J. (2019). *The deep history of ourselves: The four-billion-year history of how we got conscious brains*. New York: Viking.

Libby, E. & Rainey, P. B. (2013). A conceptual framework for the evolutionary origins of multicellularity. *Physical Biology,* 10: 1–9.

Lupien, S. J., McEwen, B. S., Gunnar, M. R., & Heim, C. (2009). Effects of stress throughout the lifespan on the brain, behaviour and cognition. *Nature Reviews/ Neuroscience,* 10: 434–445.

MacGregor, R. (1962). Multiple impact psychotherapy with families. *Family Process.* 1: 15–29.

Margulis, L. (1981). *Symbiosis in cell evolution: Life and its environment on the early earth*. San Francisco: W. H. Freeman.

Margulis, L. & Sagan, D. (2002). *Acquiring genomes: A theory of the origin of species*. New York: Basic Books.

Maslow, A. H. (1971). *The farther reaches of human nature*. New York: The Viking Press.

Mayr, E. (1982). *The growth of biological thought: Diversity, evolution, and inheritance*. Cambridge, MA: The Belknap Press of Harvard University.

McEwen, B. S. (2007). Physiology and neurobiology of stress and adaptation: Central role of the brain. *Physiological Review,* 87: 873–904.

McEwen B. S. & Gianaros, P. J. (2010). "Central role of the brain in stress and adaptation: Links to socioeconomic status, health, and disease." *Annals of the New York Academy of Sciences,* 1186: 190–222.

McEwen, B. S. & Gianaros, P. J. (2011). Stress- and allostasis- induced brain plasticity. *Annual Review of Medicine,* 62: 5.1–5.15.

McGowan, P. O. 2013. Epigenomic mechanisms of early adversity and HPA dysfunction: Considerations for PTSD research. *Frontiers in Psychiatry,* 26 September 2013, https://doi.org/103389/fpsyt.201300110, 1–6.

McKnight, A. S. (2020). Emotional cutoff. In M. Keller & R. Noone (Eds.), *Handbook of Bowen family systems theory and research methods*. New York: Routledge Press, pp. 157–173.

Meaney, M. J. (2010). Epigenetics and the biological definition of gene x environment interactions. *Child Development,* 81: 41–79.

Meaney, M. J. & Szyf, M. (2005). Maternal care as a model for experience-dependent chromatin plasticity? *TRENDS in Neurosciences,* 28: 456–463.

Merriam-Webster Dictionary. (2020). Springfield, MA.

Miller, G., Rohleder, N., & Cole, S. W. (2009). Chronic interpersonal stress predicts activation of pro- and anti-inflammatory signaling pathways six months later. *Psychosomatic Medicine,* 71: 57–62.

Narita, K., Takei, Y., Suda, M., Aoyama, Y., Uehara, T., Kosaka, H., Amanum, M., Fukuda, M., & Mikuni, M. (2010). Relationship of parental bonding styles with gray matter volume of dorsolateral prefrontal cortex in young adults. *Progress in Neuro-Psychopharmacology & Biological Psychiatry,* 34: 624–631.

Neill, J. R. & Kniskern, D. P. (1982). *From psyche to system: The evolving therapy of Carl* Whitaker. New York: The Guilford Press.

Noone, R. J. (2014). Differentiation of self as a multigenerational process. In P. Titelman (Ed.), *Differentiation of self: Bowen family systems theory perspectives.* New York: Routledge.

Noone, R. J. (2015). Multigenerational family emotional process as a source of individual differences in adaptiveness. In R. Noone & D. Papero (Eds.), *The family emotional system.* Lanham, MD: Lexington Books.

Noone, R. J. (2016). Family, self, and the intermix of emotional and intellectual functioning. *Family Systems,* 12: 29–52.

Noone, R. J. & Reddig, R. (1976). Case studies in the family treatment of drug abuse. *Family Process,* 15: 325–332.

Noone, R. J. & Papero, D. V. (2015). *The family emotional system.* Lanham, MD: Lexington Books.

Norman, G. J., Hawkley, L. C., Cole, S. W., Berntson, G. G., & Cacioppo, J. T. (2012). Social neuroscience: The social brain, oxytocin, and health. *Social Neuroscience,* 7: 18–29.

Nusslock, R. & Miller, G. E. (2016). Early life adversity and physical and emotional health across the lifespan: A neuroimmune network hypothesis. *Biological Psychiatry,* 80: 23–32.

O'Connor, T. G. & Sefair, A. V. (2019). Stress and physiology in clinical research with risk exposed children: From mechanism to application. *Adoption & Fostering,* 43: 340–350.

Panksepp, J. (1998). *Affective neuroscience: The foundations of human and animal emotions.* New York: Oxford University Press.

Papero, D. V. (1990). *Bowen family systems theory.* Boston: Allyn and Bacon.

Papero, D. V. (2015). The family emotional system. In R. Noone & D. Papero (Eds.), *The family emotional system.* Lanham, MD: Lexington Books.

Papero, D. V. (2017). Trauma and the family: A systems-oriented approach. *Australian & New Zealand Journal of Family Therapy, 38*: 582–594.

Papero, D. V. (2018). Developing a systems model for family assessment. *Family Systems,* 13: 129–144.

Papero, D. V. (2020). A systems model for family assessment. In M. Keller & R. Noone (Eds.), *Handbook of Bowen family systems theory and research methods.* New York: Routledge Press, pp. 36–45.

Papero, D. V., Frost, R. T., Havstad, L., & Noone, R. J. (2018). Natural systems thinking and the human family. *Systems,* 6: 19–29.

Pinker, S. (2011). *The better angels of our nature: Why violence has declined.* New York: Penguin Books.

Porges, S. W. (2011). *The polyvagal theory: Neurophysiological foundations of emotions, attachment, communication, and self-regulation.* New York: W.W. Norton.

Raio, C. M., Orederu, T. A., Palazzolo, L., Shurick, A. A., & Phelps, E. A. (2013). Cognitive emotion regulation fails the stress test. *PNAS,* 110: 15139–15144.

Rakow, C. (in press). The back story on developing the concept of differentiation as seen in the Murray Bowen Archives. *Family Systems.*

Repetti, R. L., Robles, T. F., & Reynolds, B. (2011). Allostatic processes in the family. *Development and Psychopathology,* 23: 921–938.

Roth, T. L. & Sweatt, J. D. (2011). Epigenetic mechanisms and environmental shaping of the brain during sensitive periods of development. *Journal of Child Psychology and Psychiatry,* 52: 398–408.

Rubenstein, D. R., Agren, J. A., Carbone, L., Elde, N. C., Hoekstra, H. E., Kapheim, K. M., Keller, L., Moreau, C. S., Toth, A. L., Yeaman, S., & Hofmann, H. A. (2019). Coevolution of genome architecture and social behavior. *Trends in Ecology and Evolution,* 34: 844–855.

Salmon, C. A. & Shackelford, T. K. (2007). *Family relationships: An evolutionary perspective.* New York: Oxford University Press.

Sapolsky, R. M. (2017). *Behave: The biology of humans at our best and worst.* New York: Penguin Press.

Sapp, J. (2003). *Genesis: The evolution of biology.* New York: Oxford University Press.

Sapp, J. (2009). *The new foundations of evolution.* New York: Oxford University Press.

Shapiro, J. A. (2011). *Evolution: A view from the 21st century.* Upper Saddle River, NJ: FT Press Science.

Shields, G. S., Moons, W. G., & Slavich, G. M. (2017a). Better executive function under stress mitigates the effects of recent life stress exposure on health in young adults. *Stress,* 20: 75–85.

Shields, G. S., Moons, W. G., & Slavich, G. M. (2017b). Inflammation, self-regulation, and health: An immunologic model of self-regulatory failure. *Perspectives in Psychological Science,* 12: 588–612.

Shonkoff, J. P., Boyce, W. T., & McEwen, B. S. (2009). Neuroscience, molecular biology, and the childhood roots of health disparities. *JAMA,* 301: 2252–2259.

Silvers, J. A., Buhle, J. T., & Ochsner, K. N. (2013). The neuroscience of emotion regulation: Basic mechanisms and their role in development, aging, and psychopathology. In K. Ochsner & S. Kosslyn (Eds.), *The Oxford Handbook of Cognitive Neuroscience, Vol I.* New York: Oxford University Press.

Slavich, G. M. & Cole, S. W. (2013). The emerging field of human social genomics. *Clinical Psychological Science.* 1: 331–348.

Snowdon, C. T. & Ziegler, T. E. (2007). Growing up cooperatively: Family processes and infant care in marmosets and tamarins. *The Journal of Developmental Processes,* 2: 40–66.

Sterling, P. & Eyer, J. (1988). Allostasis: A new paradigm to explain arousal pathology. In S. Fisher & J. Reason (Eds.), *Handbook of Life Stress, Cognition, and Health.* New York: John Wiley and Sons.

Storey, A. E. & Ziegler, T. E. (2016). Primate paternal care: Interactions between biology and social experience. *Hormones and Behavior, 77:* 260–271.

Sulloway, F. J. (1996). *Born to rebel: Birth order, family dynamics, and creative lives.* New York: Pantheon Books.

Szyf, M. (2019). The epigenetics of perinatal stress. *Dialogues in Clinical Neuroscience, 21:* 369–378.

Szyf, M., McGowan, P., & Meaney, M. J. (2008). The social environment and the epigenome. *Environmental and Molecular Mutagenesis, 49:* 46–60.

Tang, A. C., Akers, K. G., Reeb, B. C., Romeo, R. D., & McEwen, B. S. (2006). Programming social, cognitive, and neuroendocrine development by early exposure to novelty. *Proceedings of the National Academy of Sciences, 103:* 15716–15721.

Taub, D. D. (2008). Neuroendocrine interactions in the immune system. *Cell Immunology, 252:* 1–6.

Toman, W. (1969). *Family constellation: Its effects on personality and social behavior.* New York: Springer Publishing Company.

Tomasello, M. (2019). *Becoming human: A theory of ontogeny.* Cambridge, MA: The Belknap Press of Harvard University Press.

Uvnas Moberg, K. (2003). *The oxytocin factor: Tapping the hormone of calm, love, and healing.* Cambridge, MA: Da Capo Press.

Walker, C., Deschamps, S., Proul x, K., Tu, M., Salzman, C., Woodside, B., Lupien, S., Gallo-Payet, N., & Richard, D. (2004). Mother to infant or infant to mother? Reciprocal regulation of responsiveness to stress in rodents and the implications for humans. *Journal of Psychiatry and Neuroscience, 29:* 364–82.

Weaver, I. C., Cervoni, N., Champagne, F. A., D'Alessio, A. C., Sharma, S., Seckl, J. R., Dymov, S., Szyf, M., & Meaney, M. J. (2004). Epigenetic programming by maternal behavior. *Nature Neuroscience, 7:* 847–854.

West-Eberhard, M. J. (2003). *Developmental plasticity and evolution.* New York: Oxford University Press.

Wilson, D. S. (2019). *This view of life: Completing the Darwinian revolution.* New York: Vintage Books.

Wilson, E. O. (2012). *The social conquest of earth.* New York: Liveright.

Young, A. I., Benonisdottir, S., Przeworski, M., & Kong, A. (2019). Deconstructing the sources of genotype-phenotype associations in humans. *Science, 365:* 1396–1400.

Zhang, T. & Meaney, M. J. (2010). Epigenetics and the environmental regulation of the genome and its function. *Annual Review of Psychology, 61:* 439–66.

Index

Ackerman, Nathan, 160
ACTH (adrenocorticotropic hormone),
  108
acute *vs.* chronic anxiety, 112
adaptive capacity, 9–27; brain activity
  and development, 47–48, 57–58,
  198–99; Bwa Mawego population,
  106–7; decline over generations,
  123–24; detriangling self from
  emotional situations, 188–89;
  differentiation of self as central to,
  17, 19–27, 52–57, 165–66, 173–76;
  emotional process symbols, *180*;
  epigenetics in individual differences,
  164–65; evolutionary perspective,
  13–17, 39–40, 89–92, 197–200;
  as existing in all life, 66; extended
  family's contribution to, 151; family
  adaptive patterns, 70–85; family
  diagram and history, 176–79, *178–
  79*; family's influence on individual
  development, 18–19, 99, 133–34;
  as focus of mental health field, 32;
  human prospects for the future, 197–
  98; individualistic paradigm for, 10–
  15, 17–18; intellectual system, 52–
  57; multigenerational transmission as
  central to, 118, 119, 128–29, 163–64;
  nodal events, 182–83; objectivity's
  contribution to, 125; and observation
  ability, 179–81; Papero's basic
  functions, 85; parental triangle and
  expanding observation lens, 184–88;
  person-to-person relationships, 183–
  84; regulating emotional reactivity,
  68–69, 181–82; siblings, 189–90,
  190–91; societal, 162; stress's role
  in, 17, 24, 68, 71, 83–84, 105–18,
  114; and temperament, 11; variation
  in, 13–14, 17, 71; work and other
  relationship systems, 191–93. *See
  also* chronic anxiety
adaptiveness framework (Papero), 85
adaptive response, emotional cutoff as,
  138, 143–44
addiction, 60–61
adolescence: autonomy *vs.* dependence
  struggle, 135–36, 157; brain
  development during, 51, 58; in
  family projection process, 153;
  unresolved emotional attachment,
  157, 165
Adolphs, Ralph, 45–46
adrenocorticotropic hormone (ACTH),
  108
affect, evolutionary perspective, 45. *See
  also* emotions
affective neuroscience, 45

About the Author

Robert J. Noone, PhD, is faculty at the Center for Family Consultation, Evanston, IL, and the Bowen Center for the Study of the Family/Georgetown Family Center in Washington, D.C. He is the editor of the journal *Family Systems* and coeditor of the books *The Family Emotional System* (2015) and *Handbook of Bowen Family Systems Theory and Research Methods* (2020). Dr. Noone has a practice in family psychotherapy in Evanston, IL. He received his doctorate from the University of Illinois at Chicago and postgraduate training at Georgetown University Medical Center in Washington, D.C.

www.ingramcontent.com/pod-product-compliance
Lightning Source LLC
Chambersburg PA
CBHW022311280326
41932CB00010B/1056